EAT WITH
THE
*flow*

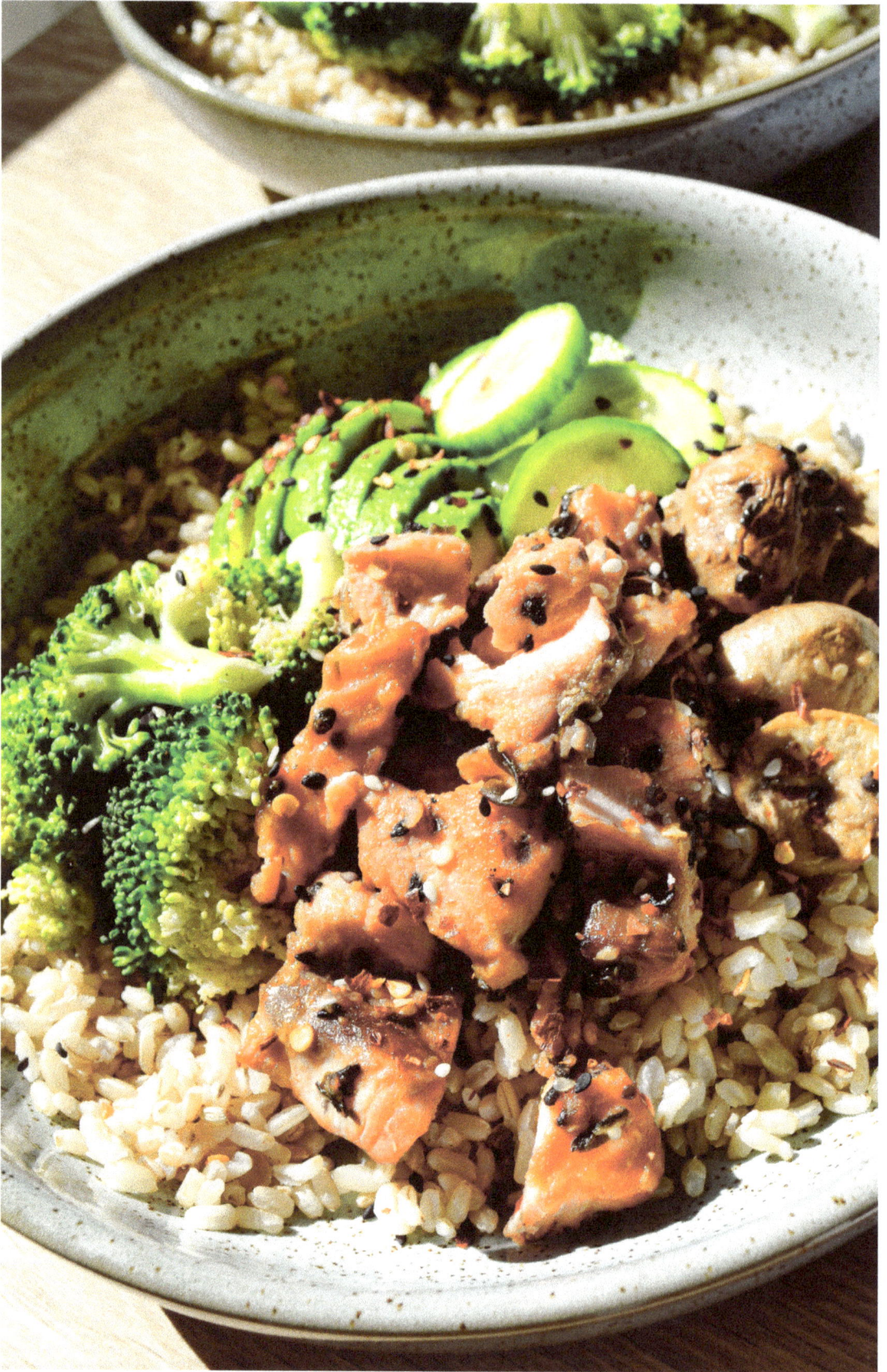

# EAT WITH THE *flow*

## RECIPES TO GET IN SYNC WITH YOUR CYCLE

## TARYN DARLOW

First published in 2025 by Dean Publishing
PO Box 119
Mt. Macedon, Victoria, 3441
Australia
deanpublishing.com

DEAN
PUBLISHING

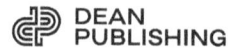

Cataloguing-in-Publication Data
National Library of Australia
Title: Eat With The Flow – Recipes To Get In Sync With Your Cycle
Edition: 1st edn
ISBN: 978-1-764372-30-5
Category: Cooking/Health & Healing

Conceptual Cover Design, Layout and Graphics: Pamela Soto
Recipe photos: Taryn Darlow & Pamela Soto
Back cover photo: Nik Epifanidis

# CONTENTS

# welcome

Welcome to *Eat With the Flow*. This book was designed and curated to support your menstrual cycle with food, so you can feel your best and thrive in every phase of your cycle.

Whether you're looking to harness the power of your hormones to feel more energised and in tune with your body or you're navigating health conditions that affect your hormones and reproductive health, *Eat With the Flow* is here to guide you.

Love Taryn

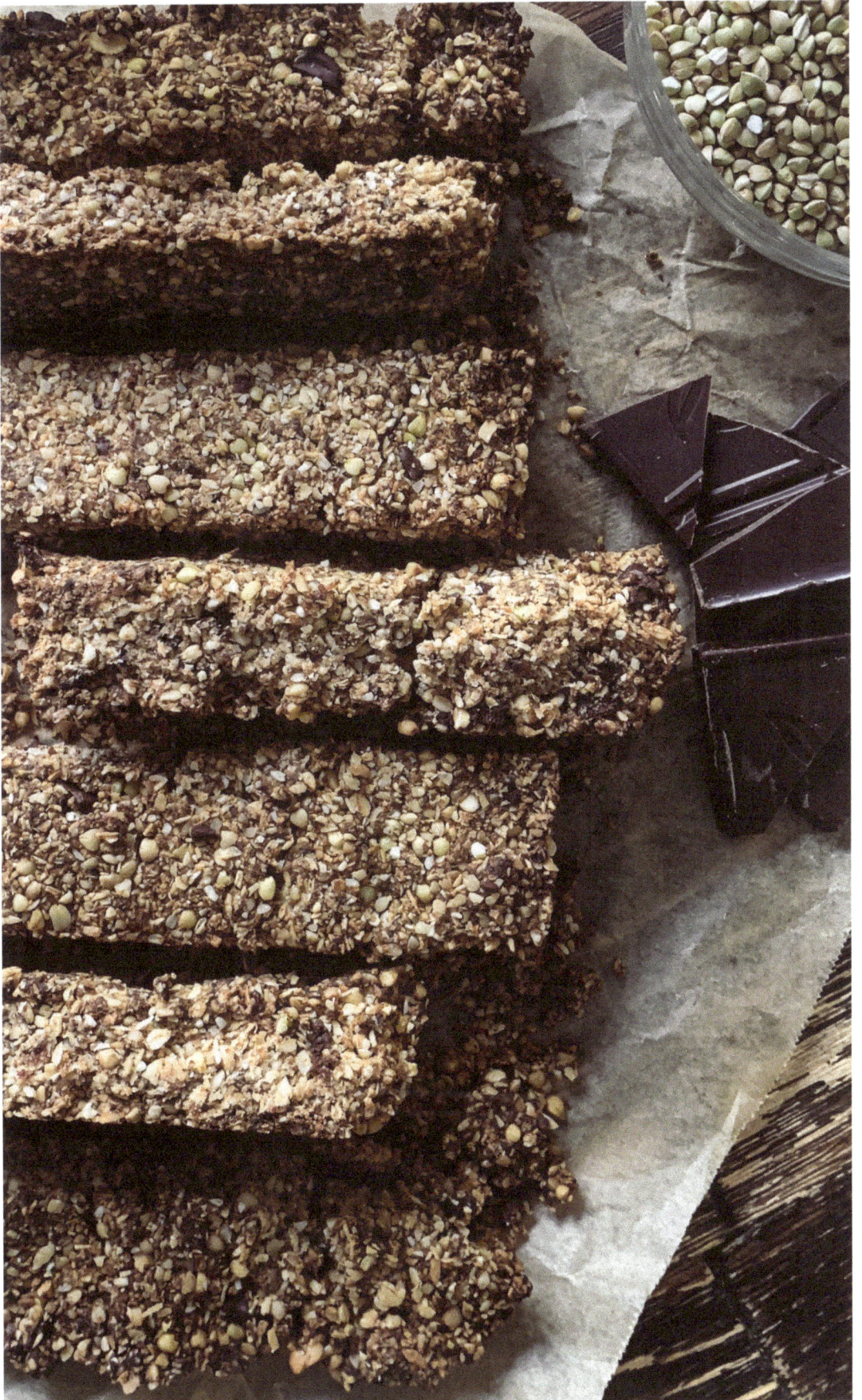

# ABOUT THE AUTHOR

For my entire young adult life, I suffered from adult acne. It wasn't just before my period, it was all the time. This significantly impacted my self confidence, but I didn't realise the effect it was also having on my health. When visiting the doctors seeking help, I was only given one option: to go on the pill (hormonal contraception). At the time, I refused. I didn't need it for contraceptive purposes and I was aware of the issues associated with cardiovascular health and stroke risks. Fast forward to today, I feel reassured to know there are always other options available.

I knew there had to be another way to heal my skin that wasn't a 'band-aid solution' like the pill or other medications. So I set out to find out how to fix my skin naturally. I soon learned about the impact of food and how foods like dairy, gluten and eggs can be inflammatory, so I began to cut these out. I saw some results with my skin clearing, but not a huge difference. Unfortunately, this obsession of avoiding certain foods, led me to develop a negative association with particular foods and forced me to not enjoy them, even in moderation. I was so fixated and fearful of consuming them that even the tiniest bit of milk or cheese caused me to break out. Little did I know that having a restrictive diet was also negatively affecting my overall health, which I will talk about later in this section. It may have been the food, but it was most likely the stress and manifestation of breakouts that was causing the acne. I started to develop a negative attitude towards food for the first time in my life, and I was not okay with the beliefs that were building.

While trying to heal my skin on the inside, I worked on healing it from the outside too. I followed a specific routine both morning and night and used high quality products, which helped me to clear my skin at the surface, unblocking the pores and managing the oiliness. Although this helped a lot, I was still experiencing breakouts during ovulation and menstruation. The healing process was quicker with the products but I still hadn't managed to get to the root cause to stop the hormonal imbalance happening internally that was showing up externally.

## Why I Created This Book

Since my acne was now only flaring up around ovulation and menstruation, I started to delve into what exactly happens to our bodies throughout our cycle. This led me down a rabbit hole of research, experimentation and transformation. The intricate balance of hormones and the phases of the menstrual cycle influence not just our reproductive health but our overall wellbeing. After years of learning and testing, I was able to sync my diet and exercise to my cycle, leading to clear, glowing skin and a body that felt good most of the time. This new way of living soon became 'gospel' to me.

I wanted to help others in the same way I helped myself, so I went on to study women's health and nutrition coaching with WellCollege, fertility and menstrual cycle

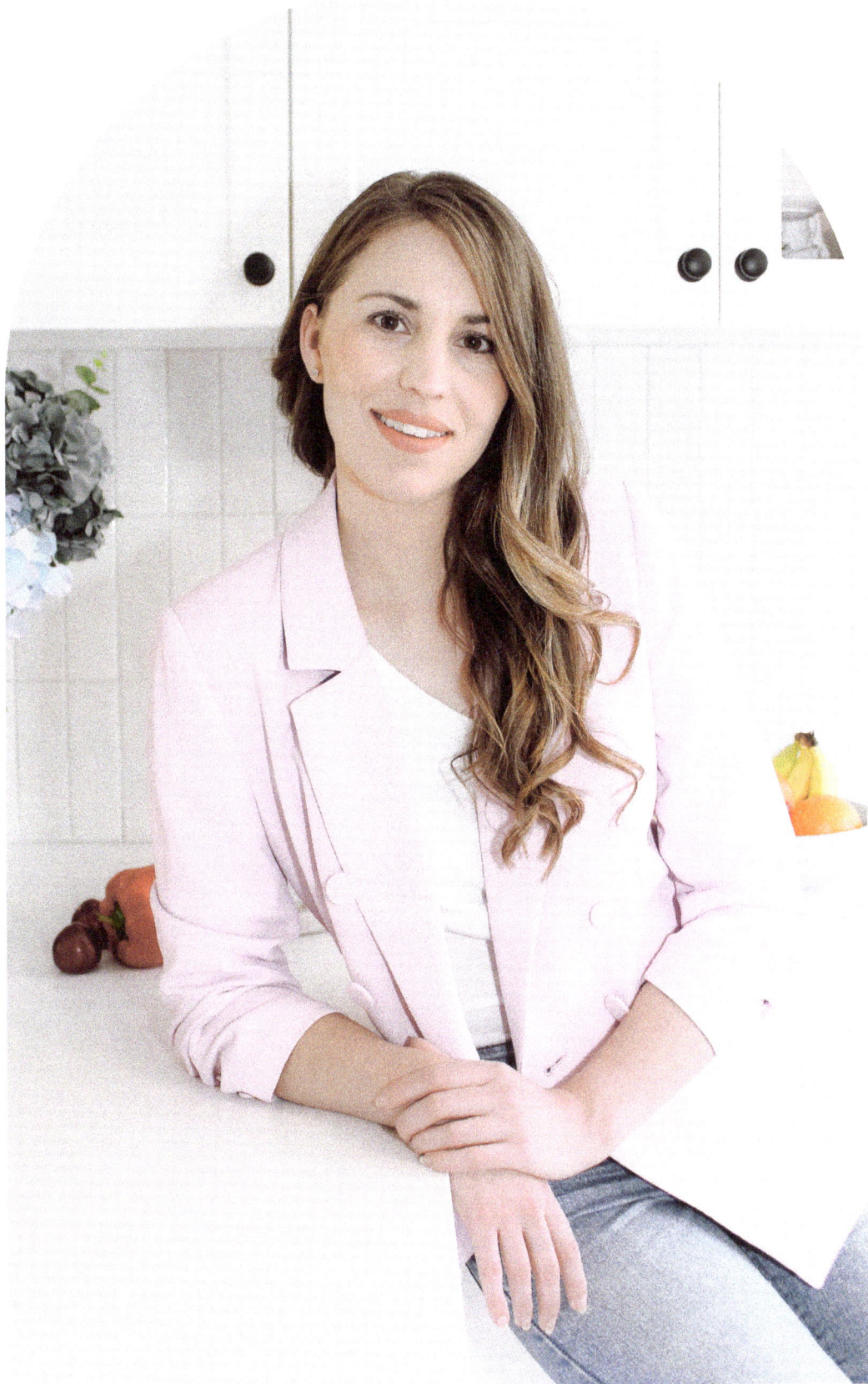

education with FEMM (Fertility Education & Medical Management), and Female Fundamentals™ with Dr Anthea Todd. I also became certified as a practitioner in hair tissue mineral analysis with Interclinical Laboratories and became a coach and practitioner in neurolinguistic programming, quantum healing and breathwork with

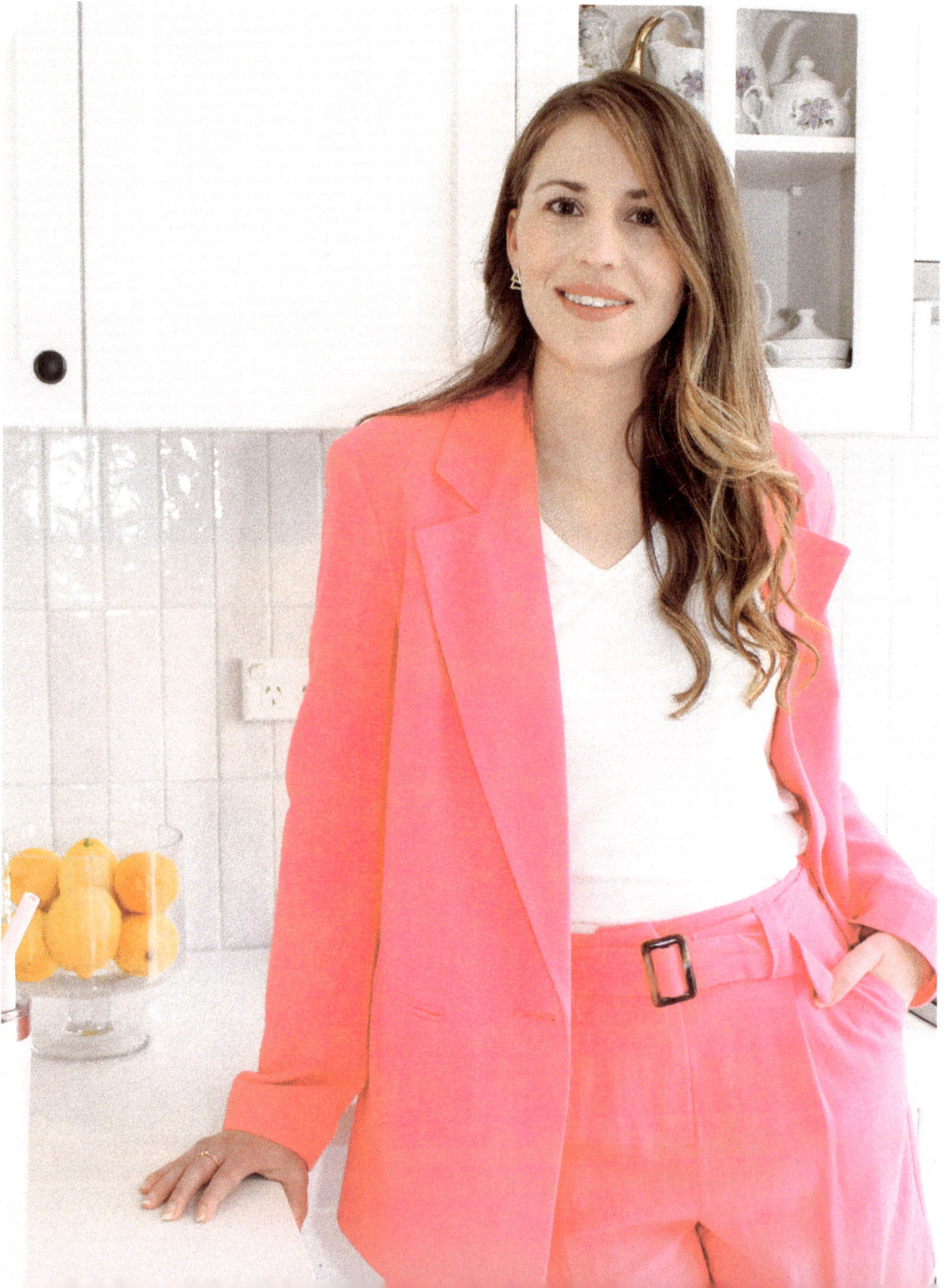

Elizabeth Anne Walker. I combined all my knowledge from the abundance of books I have read for my own healing, along with the knowledge in my training to produce the best quality cookbook for you and your health that I can.

I initially just created this book for myself; however, I realised it needed to be shared with the world and I needed to do more to help others. This book is a tailored guide to support you through the journey of your cycle. Understanding the delicate balance of hormones and their profound impact on your body allows you to make informed choices, especially in regards to nutrition.

As you delve into the recipes and nutritional insights in the following chapters, remember that food is not merely sustenance; it's a powerful ally in fostering health, vitality and longevity. The landmark Harvard Nurses' Study underscores the significant role nutrition plays in fertility and menstrual health, reaffirming that food is nature's medicine.

I firmly believe in the transformative power of nourishing your body, and that belief is the driving force behind this book. By aligning your dietary choices with the ebbs and flows of your menstrual cycle, you can embark on a journey of holistic wellbeing. Whether you have a natural cycle, are on hormonal birth control or face irregularities, these recipes are designed to cater to and support your unique nutritional needs, by simply providing you with well-balanced meals.

This is not a diet book. This is a framework for nourishment. The recipes in this book have been thoughtfully crafted with your hormones in mind and designed to support your body's changing needs throughout the menstrual cycle. But this isn't about rigid rules or 'perfect' eating. Instead, it's a gentle guide to help you tune in to your body, choose meals that feel nourishing and develop a deeper connection with your cyclical nature. As each recipe is complete, with protein, fats and carbohydrates to support blood sugar and hormone balance, you can trust that whatever you choose, whenever you choose it, will serve your health. If a comforting meal from the menstrual phase calls to you during ovulation, lean in. Your body knows what it needs, and this book is here to help you honour that.

So, let's embark on this culinary journey together, celebrating each phase of your cycle and embracing the profound connection between what you eat and how you feel. Remember, nourishing your body appropriately is not just a good choice; it's a path to flourishing and living your healthiest, happiest life.

You can also join me at Flo.urish by Taryn on socials to further educate and empower yourself to improve your hormone health, menstrual health and overall fertility.

# THE MENSTRUAL CYCLE

*The menstrual cycle is a complex, natural
process controlled by the sex hormones and
regulated by a variety of other hormones.
The menstrual cycle can be broken down into
four phases: menstrual, follicular, ovulation
and luteal. To best understand the menstrual
cycle, it is helpful to know about the major sex
hormones that influence it.*

# Hormones of the Menstrual Cycle

## Follicle Stimulating Hormone (FSH)

FSH is produced and released by the pituitary gland, which is located in the brain. This hormone stimulates follicles in the ovary and causes them to grow, mature, and eventually be released during ovulation. The development of the follicle results in the production and release of oestrogen.

## Oestrogen

Oestrogen is the female sex hormone. There are three types of oestrogens in the body and they are responsible for growth and development in the body. The main form of oestrogen is produced in the ovaries, while the other two are produced from testosterone and in the adrenal glands.

In the menstrual cycle, oestrogen stimulates the thickening of the endometrium (uterine lining), causes the cervix to release mucus that is slippery, clear and abundant, and is involved in ovulation. As oestrogen is a steroid hormone, it is responsible for building breast, fat and liver tissue, forming bones, improving insulin sensitivity, creating and stimulating brain cells, promoting blood clotting and protecting against heart disease.

## Luteinising Hormone (LH)

LH is released by the pituitary gland when oestrogen reaches a sufficient level, which triggers the egg to be released from the ovary. After ovulation, LH transforms the follicle into the corpus luteum, which will produce progesterone.

## Progesterone

Progesterone is produced by the newly transformed follicle, the corpus luteum in the ovary, after ovulation occurs. It is the 'maintainer' in the body. Its role within the menstrual cycle is to maintain the health of the uterine lining to ensure it is ready for the implantation of a fertilised egg. Progesterone helps to relax the uterus, maintain bone density and health, relax blood vessels, increase insulin resistance, maintain and heal brain cells, promote sleep and relaxation, and decrease anxiety. Progesterone is only produced if ovulation occurs.

## Testosterone

Testosterone is a type of androgen and its role in the menstrual cycle is to support the ovary to release an egg at ovulation. Testosterone is responsible for increasing libido, improving confidence and motivation and building muscle. Testosterone also converts into oestrogen, specifically estrone. Testosterone in women is in smaller amounts in comparison to men.

# Other Hormones that Influence the Menstrual Cycle

## Cortisol

Cortisol is a hormone produced and released by the adrenal glands (which sit on top of your kidneys). It's not only released in response to stress but also to support essential functions such as reducing inflammation, regulating blood glucose, and aiding in growth and development. Cortisol levels naturally fluctuate throughout the day, peaking in the early morning to help you wake up and reaching their lowest levels at night to support rest and recovery. However, when the body experiences ongoing or excessive stress, cortisol production increases. Chronically elevated cortisol can disrupt hormonal balance because cortisol and the sex hormones share the same building block: cholesterol. During periods of stress, the body prioritises producing cortisol over sex hormones to manage the stress response, as survival always takes precedence over reproduction.

## Insulin

Insulin is a hormone produced and released by the pancreas in response to rising blood glucose levels after eating. When food is broken down into glucose and absorbed into the bloodstream, the pancreas releases insulin to help move glucose from the blood into the body's cells where it can be used for energy. The amount of insulin released depends on how much glucose is present in the blood. Acting as a 'gatekeeper', insulin facilitates this process and helps regulate blood sugar levels within a healthy range.

The regulation of blood sugars is interdependent of stress and the nervous system. Beyond blood sugar regulation, insulin also plays a significant role in sex hormone balance. When insulin levels remain consistently high, due to excessive sugar or refined carbohydrate intake, or due to inconsistent eating patterns, the body can become insulin resistant, meaning the cells no longer respond effectively to insulin. This leads to higher circulating insulin levels, which can disrupt hormonal balance. In women, excess insulin stimulates the ovaries to produce more androgens, such as testosterone, contributing to conditions like polycystic ovary syndrome (PCOS). It can also interfere with ovulation and disrupt the balance of estrogen and progesterone, impacting menstrual cycle regularity and fertility.

## Sex Hormone Binding Globulin (SHBG)

SHBG is a hormone that controls the amount of sex-hormones (oestrogen and testosterone) that are roaming free in the bloodstream. The body makes oestrogen and testosterone, and SHBG keeps these hormones restrained until they are needed to ensure they are balanced in the body. Should other hormones, like insulin, be out of balance, it impacts the balance of the SHBG, and consequently other hormones as well.

# The Phases of the Menstrual Cycle

The menstrual cycle consists of four distinct phases: menstrual, follicular, ovulatory, and luteal. While these are commonly referred to as separate stages, they fall under two broader phases: follicular (which includes the menstrual, follicular and ovulatory phases) and the luteal phase. These phases are regulated by hormonal changes throughout the course of the cycle. During the menstrual cycle, two cycles are occurring at the same time: the ovarian cycle, which focuses on activity in the ovaries (like follicle development and ovulation), and the endometrial cycle, which describes the changes in the uterine lining in preparation for a possible pregnancy. For the purpose of this book, the menstrual cycle will be broken up into the four phases across a 28-day cycle. Cycle lengths vary from person to person though and will typically be between 21–35 days.

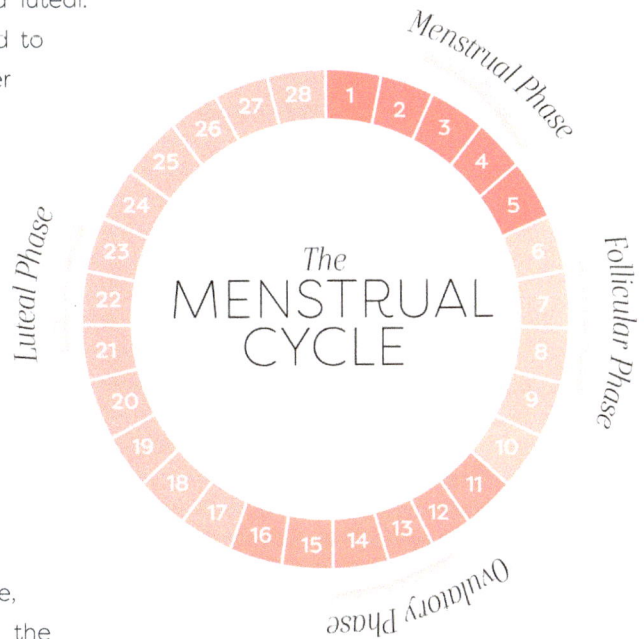

The
## MENSTRUAL CYCLE

Menstrual Phase

Follicular Phase

Ovulatory Phase

Luteal Phase

## The Menstrual Phase

The menstrual phase marks the beginning of a new cycle and occurs when the uterine lining (endometrium) that was developing in the previous cycle begins to shed. This is known as the period (menstrual bleeding). It occurs as a result of the egg not being fertilised. A healthy menstrual phase lasts between 3-7 days, with at least one day of moderate to heavy bleeding (indicating sufficient levels of oestrogen). During this phase, the hormone levels, particularly oestrogen and progesterone are low, with FSH beginning to rise to prepare the next follicle. The rise in FSH also causes menstruation to stop.

### The Follicular Phase

The follicular phase is the time between menstruation and ovulation. During this phase, the pituitary gland in the brain releases follicle stimulating hormone (FSH), which communicates with the ovary to stimulate the development of several follicles (which contain an egg) in the ovary. The development of these follicles cause them to produce and release oestrogen, causing the uterine lining to thicken. Over a few days, the most mature and dominant follicle will continue to develop, which will be the egg that is released in ovulation.

### Ovulatory Phase

The ovulatory phase is when the egg ruptures from the follicle and is released into the fallopian tube. Ovulation occurs when oestrogen has reached its peak, or a sufficient amount, causing the sudden spike of luteinising hormone (LH) and triggering the follicle to release the egg. This is the 'main event' of the menstrual cycle and generally occurs at the mid-point of the cycle. The timing of ovulation can fluctuate from month to month.

## HORMONES THROUGH THE MENSTRUAL CYCLE

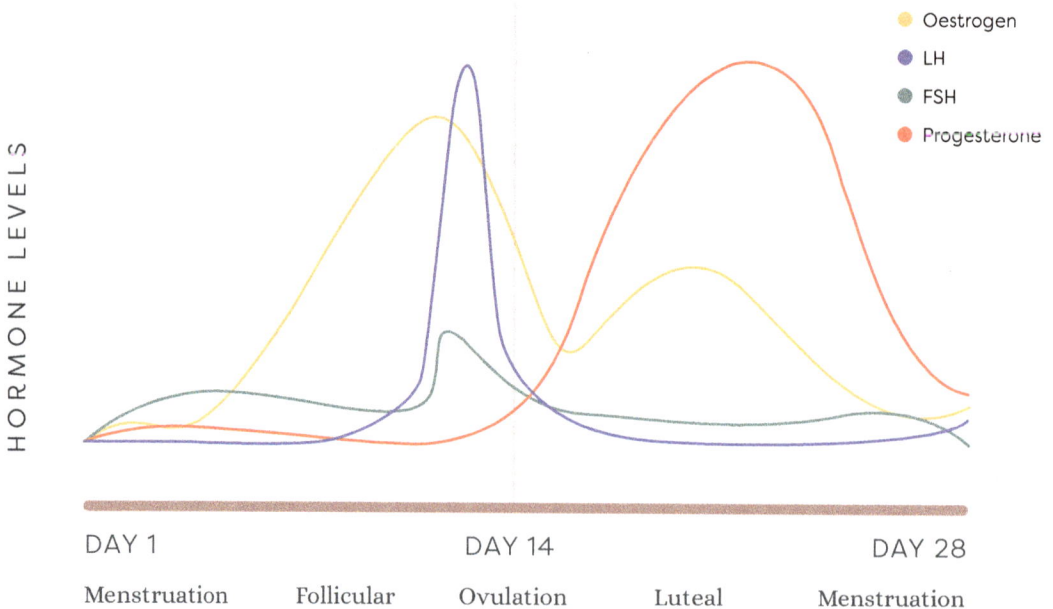

Legend: Oestrogen, LH, FSH, Progesterone

HORMONE LEVELS

DAY 1 — Menstruation
Follicular
DAY 14 — Ovulation
Luteal
DAY 28 — Menstruation

The Phases of the Menstrual Cycle

## Luteal Phase

The final phase of the cycle begins after ovulation and lasts for 9–18 days, depending on the individual's cycle length. During this phase, progesterone released by the corpus luteum (the former follicle), causes the uterine lining to continue to thicken, preparing for the possible implantation of a fertilised egg.

After about 5 days, if the uterine lining receives fertilised egg and implantation occurs, a hormone called hCG (human chorionic gonadotropin) will tell the corpus luteum to continue producing progesterone to support the pregnancy until the placenta can take over.

However, if it doesn't receive a fertilised egg, the corpus luteum will begin to break down and progesterone production will stop. This drop in progesterone causes the endometrium to break down, which results in a period in the following days. This leads to the start of the menstrual phase and the cycle beginning again.

# Influences of the Menstrual Cycle

There are over 50 hormones in the body, each responsible for controlling and regulating essential functions. When any of these hormones are out of balance, our body cannot perform at its best. Reproductive and menstrual health is deeply interconnected with overall health – when one is disrupted, the other is affected.

Many factors influence menstrual cycle health, including but not limited to metabolism, thyroid function, adrenal health, sleep, liver function, blood glucose regulation, body weight, gut health, nutrient deficiencies, and environmental toxins. This section will explore how each of these impacts reproductive health.

## Thyroid Health

The thyroid is a gland in the endocrine system that produces hormones to regulate numerous bodily functions, including the menstrual cycle. An underactive thyroid (hypothyroidism) can lead to irregular, heavy, or absent periods, along with fatigue, weight gain, and cold intolerance. An overactive thyroid (hyperthyroidism) can result in shorter, lighter, or infrequent periods, as well as symptoms like nervousness, weight loss, and heat intolerance. Thyroid dysfunction can also affect fertility by preventing ovulation or impacting egg quality. Imbalances in key minerals like selenium, magnesium, calcium and zinc can impair thyroid function, hormone production and conversion. Magnesium supports the conversion of thyroid hormones into active forms, while selenium protects the thyroid from inflammation and oxidative stress.

## Stress and Adrenal Health

The adrenal glands produce cortisol and small amounts of sex hormones such as oestrogen, progesterone and testosterone. Since all these hormones are made from cholesterol, chronic stress leads to the prioritisation of cortisol production at the expense of reproductive hormones. This can result in irregular cycles, delayed ovulation, PMS symptoms, and insulin imbalances, further affecting menstrual health. Additionally, undereating (particularly protein), fasting and diets that eliminate certain macronutrients place the body under stress, leading

to further disruptions in hormone production and cycle regulation.

## Sleep

Sleep is essential for hormonal balance. Progesterone promotes sleep, but disruptions in progesterone levels – along with imbalances in cortisol, melatonin, and insulin – can lead to poor sleep quality. Since sleep is a time for replenishment and restoration, insufficient sleep prevents hormones from being properly regulated, leading to further imbalances. Optimal sleep depends on sufficient levels of magnesium, calcium, and sodium, which calm the nervous system and support melatonin production. Deficiencies in these minerals can contribute to insomnia, night waking, and restless sleep, which impact the body's ability to restore and recharge.

## Liver Health

The liver plays a key role in detoxification, including the metabolism and excretion of excess hormones, particularly oestrogen. If the liver is not functioning optimally, oestrogen dominance can occur, leading to heavy or painful periods, PMS symptoms, low libido, bloating, fatigue, anxiety, and conditions such as endometriosis and fibroids. The liver relies on magnesium, zinc, copper, sulfur and molybdenum for detoxification, hormone clearance and enzyme function. Sulfur-rich compounds and molybdenum are essential for phase two liver detox pathways, supporting the safe breakdown and elimination of excess hormones like oestrogen.

## Body Weight
Body weight and menstrual cycle health are closely linked. Low body weight can decrease oestrogen production, disrupting ovulation and causing irregular cycles. Excess body weight, on the other hand, can lead to high oestrogen levels, contributing to menstrual irregularities. Additionally, excess weight can increase insulin resistance, further impacting hormone balance. Minerals like zinc, chromium, and magnesium support insulin sensitivity, metabolism, and appetite regulation. Imbalances can contribute to weight gain, blood sugar imbalances and disrupted hormone production.

## Blood Glucose Regulation
Blood glucose regulation plays a critical role in hormone balance. Oestrogen increases insulin sensitivity, while progesterone decreases it. If blood sugar levels are imbalanced, hormones will be too. Insulin resistance, often caused by excessive sugar intake, frequent blood sugar spikes and a dysregulated nervous system, can interfere with ovulation and reduce progesterone production, leading to irregular cycles and fertility issues. Stable blood sugar relies on calcium, magnesium, chromium, manganese, potassium and zinc. These minerals help transport glucose into cells,

regulate insulin, and reduce cravings and hormonal fluctuations tied to blood sugar highs and lows.

## A Note on PCOS and Insulin
Polycystic Ovarian Syndrome (PCOS) is a common reproductive condition driven by insulin resistance. High insulin levels suppress sex hormone-binding globulin (SHBG), increasing testosterone levels, which can lead to symptoms such as hirsutism, acne, and weight gain. It is important to note that PCOS can also be a result of stress and exhausted adrenals, coming off the pill (post-pill PCOS), inflammation and immunity.

## Gut Health
The gut microbiome is critical for hormone balance. The estrobolome, a collection of gut bacteria, metabolises and regulates oestrogen levels. Poor gut health can lead to oestrogen imbalances, contributing to menstrual health issues and increasing the risk of reproductive conditions such as PCOS and endometriosis. Gut health depends on a delicate balance of minerals like sodium, potassium, magnesium and zinc, which are essential for maintaining a healthy intestinal lining, motility, and microbial balance. These minerals also support the production of stomach acid, which is crucial for breaking down food and absorbing nutrients, including the very minerals that support menstrual health.

## Environmental Toxins and Hormone Imbalances

In today's world, exposure to environmental toxins, such as heavy metals and endocrine-disrupting chemicals, can mimic or interfere with hormone function. Many toxins deplete essential minerals, leading to imbalances that disrupt the menstrual cycle. Toxic burden can be reduced though by supporting the body through proper nutrition, ensuring adequate mineral intake, consuming a diverse diet for gut health, and optimising detox pathways (such as the liver and kidneys of the lymphatic system). By strengthening the body's ability to clear harmful substances, we can improve hormone function and menstrual cycle health. Toxins like heavy metals displace and deplete calcium, magnesium, zinc and selenium, which are minerals essential for detox, antioxidant protection and hormone regulation. Replenishing these helps reduce toxic load and protect hormone balance.

## Emotions and Menstrual Health

Our thoughts and emotions directly impact biological functions, including stress responses, immunity and neurochemical processes. In traditional Chinese medicine, the Bao Mai connection links the heart and uterus, emphasising the relationship between emotional well-being and reproductive health. Managing emotions can significantly improve menstrual health.

# NUTRITION FOR YOUR CYCLE

*Many of the factors affecting menstrual health, thyroid function, gut health, sleep, stress, weight, and blood glucose regulation, can be supported through proper nutrition. Food is one of the most accessible and powerful tools we have to nourish hormonal health and restore balance.*

The recipes in this book are designed to be complete and balanced, ensuring they provide all three macronutrients (protein, carbohydrates, and fats), which play essential roles in hormone production:

## FATS

Necessary for the production of lipid-based hormones such as oestrogen, progesterone, and androgens. Cholesterol is also a precursor to hormones like aldosterone, which helps regulate blood pressure, electrolyte balance, and fluid retention.

## PROTEIN

Crucial for the synthesis of thyroid hormones (T3 & T4), neurotransmitters (dopamine, serotonin, and melatonin), and reproductive-related hormones like gonadotropin-releasing hormone (GnRH), prolactin, insulin, and sex hormone-binding globulin (SHBG).

## CARBOHYDRATES

Essential for the production of luteinising hormone (LH), follicle stimulating hormone (FSH), and thyroid stimulating hormone (TSH).

A groundbreaking study by Harvard Nurses' Health, which followed over 18,000 participants for eight years, found that dietary choices significantly impact fertility and menstrual health. The study highlighted the importance of including specific foods while avoiding others to optimise reproductive health.

When I first started aligning my lifestyle to my cycle, it was early days and women were sharing anecdotal evidence of how it was working for them and improving their overall health and wellness.

However, research that suggests women who align their lifestyle with their cycle report greater emotional awareness, less stress, and improved body satisfaction is emerging more and more. The study also reported that women who aligned their movement and nutrition to their cycle consistently for at least three months saw improvements in various physical experiences and symptoms associated with their menstrual cycle including bloating, fatigue, food cravings and issues with eating habits. Women who aligned lifestyle to their cycle for longer (i.e., 6 months or longer) had even higher improved outcomes in their health and wellness.

## Why Does Syncing Your Nutrition Work?

Minerals, which are naturally occurring elements and compounds, are often referred to as the 'spark plugs' of the body, because they are essential for human health. Minerals are obtained through our diet and are responsible for every action and reaction in the body (metabolism). They influence energy production, hormone synthesis, brain and nerve conduction, muscle function, digestion, detoxification and more. Every function that happens in the body is influenced by minerals. This means that minerals play a significant role in the influence of hormone production and regulation, ovarian function, endometrium development and breakdown that occur throughout the menstrual cycle. Since we get minerals from the food we eat, choosing foods rich in specific minerals and timing their intake to align with the different phases of the menstrual cycle not only nourishes your body but also enhances the key physiological processes that occur in each phase of the menstrual cycle.

# Changing Hormones Means a Changing Plate

Your body needs the right minerals to have a healthy menstrual cycle. Due to the hormone fluctuations that occur throughout your menstrual cycle, your nutritional needs change as well. Therefore, when you provide your body with what it needs throughout your cycle, you'll experience a healthier menstrual cycle and improved reproductive health.

## Menstrual Phase

During the menstrual phase, your oestrogen and progesterone levels are at their lowest as your body is shedding the uterine lining. Your metabolism slows, so your caloric needs are slightly lower; however, your body is losing key minerals including iron, zinc and magnesium. Replenishing iron during the menstrual phase is vital for ensuring the oxygenation of blood so that bodily functions can be carried out sufficiently and with ease. This is particularly important for the ovaries and uterus, as they rely on consistent and sufficient oxygen supply for follicle maturation and fertilisation to occur.

During the menstrual phase, consuming zinc is beneficial due to its impact on inflammation, which will support the body and reduce oxidative stress, cramps and fatigue during this phase. Consuming magnesium during the menstrual phase is also highly beneficial as it relaxes muscles and regulates prostaglandins, resulting in fewer uterine cramps. It also supports neuromuscular function, which can be impaired due to the brain adjusting to the drop in hormones in this phase, reducing fatigue, headaches and irritability. The recipes for the menstrual phase will focus on replenishing iron, vitamin C, zinc and magnesium. These recipes will be warm and grounding foods with protein, healthy fats and slow-burning carbs to nourish your body, help ease fatigue, and compensate for the low energy and hormone levels at this time.

## Follicular Phase

As oestrogen begins to rise in the follicular phase, your energy increases, your blood sugar stabilises and your cravings decrease, but your metabolism stays relatively slow. During this phase, key vitamins and minerals like zinc, calcium, selenium and B-vitamins play an important role. Zinc helps the body make follicle stimulating hormone (FSH), which plays a role in the development of the follicle that will release the egg at ovulation and produce the oestrogen necessary for building the endometrial lining in the uterus. During the follicular phase, calcium influences the healthy development of the follicles and egg maturation. It is also vital for the production and synthesis of oestrogen, the dominant hormone in

this phase. Selenium is necessary in the follicular phase as it is responsible for thyroid function, indirectly affecting the menstrual cycle, protecting the follicles from oxidative stress and supporting hormone regulation. B-vitamins support DNA synthesis and cell division, which is essential in the development of the follicles, as well as the regulation of oestrogen metabolism and the lowering of prolactin, which if out of balance, will disturb ovulation later in the cycle.

Recipes in this phase will have nutrient-dense foods that support follicle development, detox pathways and gut health. These recipes will focus on hero ingredients like fibre-rich vegetables, fermented foods, B vitamins and key minerals like zinc, selenium and molybdenum to support liver detox of oestrogen and fuel ovulation. Cruciferous vegetables like broccoli will help clear excess oestrogen, while leafy greens and citrus support detox and cell energy. These recipes will be light and fresh, like salads, stir-fries and vibrant bowls.

## Ovulatory Phase

Oestrogen peaks during the ovulatory phase and a surge in the luteinising hormone (LH) triggers ovulation. Your metabolism is still low, meaning you require less calories and blood sugar remains stable. Due to high levels of oestrogen, choosing the right foods will ensure it remains balanced so that symptoms of oestrogen dominance, like acne and bloating, can be avoided or significantly reduced. In this phase, key vitamins and minerals, including zinc, calcium, fibre and omega-3s, are essential. Zinc supports the body's production of LH, which is required for triggering ovulation, ensuring ovulation occurs on time. Calcium is required as it interacts with oestrogen to ensure the continuous development of the endometrium, and it is necessary for the healthy rupturing of the follicle. Calcium also influences the release of gonadotropin-releasing hormone (GnRH), by stimulating the release of LH.

High fibre foods during the ovulatory phase help the body to clear excess oestrogen by binding to the hormone in the gut, which will reduce symptoms of oestrogen dominance. Omega-3 fatty acids in this phase will provide anti-inflammatory effects and support the rupturing of the follicle, leading to ovulation. Recipes in the ovulation phase focus on foods rich in antioxidants and minerals, colourful fruits and veggies, seeds, fish, and leafy greens. They will also be light and fresh with lots of raw ingredients to support digestion and detoxification of excess oestrogen.

## Luteal Phase

After ovulation, progesterone rises and your metabolism speeds up. You burn more calories at rest and may experience increased hunger or cravings, especially for carbohydrates and comfort foods. Blood sugar becomes less sensitive due to the effects of progesterone, making stabilising meals essential. In this phase, key vitamins and minerals include calcium, zinc, iron, magnesium and B-vitamins along with fibre and complex carbohydrate-rich foods. Calcium plays an integral role at this stage, as it influences sets off a series of triggers that will end up with an endometrial lining that is prepared for a fertilised egg and a successful embryo implantation. Calcium also plays a role in keeping balanced serotonin and dopamine levels, which can reduce PMS symptoms like irritability and depression. Lastly, calcium regulates muscle contraction and fluid balance, easing cramps and bloating.

Consuming magnesium rich foods in the luteal phase is particularly beneficial as it is protective against symptoms such as cramping, fluid retention, breast tenderness, fatigue and mood disturbances. It is also essential for the health of the endometrial lining, ensuring it is healthy and nutrient dense in the event of fertilisation occurring at ovulation. During this phase, zinc reduces inflammation and oxidative stress, and it also balances progesterone receptor activity, which influences mood-related neurotransmitters such as serotonin and dopamine, supporting mood shifts during PMS. B-Vitamins support the production of progesterone and stabilise blood sugar levels and mood, while fibre-rich foods continue to support the body to clear excess oestrogen in storage from the previous phases.

# Changing Hormones Means a Changing Plate

Consuming complex carbohydrates in this phase will support healthy energy levels, since oestrogen is low along with energy. Complex carbohydrates will also help stabilise serotonin and dopamine to help avoid mood swings. Recipes in this phase will ensure the replenishment of magnesium, calcium, B vitamins, fibre. These recipes will be warm and grounding meals with complex carbs, quality protein and healthy fats to keep your mood steady and energy stable. This is the most demanding phase nutritionally, so supporting your body here helps ease PMS, supports progesterone and sets you up better for the following cycle.

When you eat in alignment with your menstrual cycle, it won't only make you feel good and experience better health outcomes, but it will also ensure the support of your hormones all cycle long. Each phase lays the foundation for the next, so how you nourish your body on one day impacts the next. Consistently eating in alignment with your cycle allows you to work with your hormones and not against them. This way of eating helps to balance your hormones, boost fertility, reduce PMS, and improve your mood, energy and overall wellbeing.

## HTMA: Understanding Your Mineral Profile

If you want to take your health a step further, you can explore your unique mineral profile through Hair Tissue Mineral Analysis (HTMA). Minerals play a crucial role in hormone production, nervous system function, blood sugar regulation, metabolism, and digestive health. A HTMA test can help identify root causes of reproductive and menstrual health issues, such as imbalances in the thyroid, adrenal function, gut health and metabolism.

I offer personalised HTMA testing and coaching to help you understand your body's mineral status and make targeted nutritional changes to support your cycle. Through this, we can uncover hidden imbalances and create a tailored approach to your health. You can visit my website/instagram page for more details about this.

# How to Use This Book

The recipes in this book are for anyone to cook, eat and enjoy. However, they are tailored in a way to best support those who menstruate. This works no matter what your cycle currently looks like, whether you have a natural cycle, are on hormonal birth control or have an irregular cycle.

For people with regular cycles, the recipes in this book will help to maintain the balance but also reduce symptoms, improve overall health, and manage energy and mood levels. Those on birth control or who have irregular cycles can still benefit from this book, as the recipes are balanced, complete and nutrient rich. For those on hormonal birth control, key nutrients such as B-vitamins, vitamin C, magnesium and zinc become depleted, so eating the recipes outlined in this book will nourish your body with the right foods. For those with irregular cycles, it will provide your body with the nutrients it needs to support the hormone production and release, which can help balance hormones and regulate the menstrual cycle. For reproductive conditions like PCOS, following these recipes will be particularly beneficial as most recipes include whole-food ingredients with no inflammatory ingredients that often worsen symptoms of PCOS. Each recipe also contains all macronutrients essential for hormone production. In nourishing your body appropriately, you will be able to flourish and live your healthiest and happiest life.

It is important to know where you are in your cycle in order to do this best. This will be easiest for those with a regular cycle, yet still possible for those on hormonal birth control or with irregular cycles.

## Tracking Your Cycle on Hormonal Birth Control

The easiest way is to identify your menstrual phase through the symptoms/signs your body still gets and eat according to the recipes in the menstrual phase chapter. Once menstruation has finished, begin consuming recipes in the follicular phase chapter and do so for the next 5–10 days (depending on the length of your cycle). Following this, you can start eating for your ovulation phase for around 5 days. Finally, your luteal phase is the longest and you can begin eating the foods and recipes outlined in the luteal phase chapter after ovulation has occurred and do so until your next period arrives.

Understanding your biomarkers, which are body clues, will help you best understand each phase of your cycle as well as understand your overall hormone health. If you need help doing this, you can access courses and coaching programs with me.

## Personalisation

While this book is designed to nourish most menstruating women with whole, balanced foods, it's important to remember that every body is unique and some health conditions may benefit from extra adjustments.

For example, women with Polycystic Ovary Syndrome (PCOS) or endometriosis (endo) may find that moderating certain foods helps reduce inflammation and balance hormones more easily. Greek yoghurt is included in many recipes, as it's a great source of protein, calcium, probiotics and naturally low GI, which helps keep blood sugar stable (a big plus for PCOS). However, dairy can be mucus-forming or inflammatory for some people, potentially worsening symptoms in endometriosis or triggering excess insulin activity in PCOS.

Likewise, calcium stimulates oestrogen production which, for some women with endometriosis, may contribute to the growth of more endometrial tissue and worsen pain or PMS if not balanced well. But again, this is highly individual and fermented dairy like Greek yoghurt is often much better tolerated than other dairy types.

Some people with endo or histamine sensitivity may also find that certain vegetables and fruits, like tomatoes, capsicum, eggplant, chilli, spinach, avocado, strawberries, citrus or fermented foods like sauerkraut and miso, can trigger bloating, pain or inflammation. These foods are healthy for many but can be worth moderating or swapping if you notice flare ups.

If you suspect you react poorly to dairy or certain fruits and vegetables, you can easily reduce, omit or swap them out and test how you feel. This book is a flexible framework, not a rigid rulebook. The same goes for red meat, which provides valuable iron and zinc (essential for the menstrual phase), but may be best enjoyed in moderation for those with endo or PCOS if inflammation is a concern. Always trust your body's feedback, seek advice from your healthcare professional and feel free to adapt any recipe to your unique needs.

## A Note on Hero Ingredients

Regarding the recipes themselves, it is important to avoid substituting the hero ingredients that are listed at the start of each chapter, as they have been chosen for the vitamins, minerals and nutrients they provide. However, if you need to substitute more minor ingredients (e.g., omitting garlic and onion to make a recipe low FODMAP or substituting ingredients to make the recipe vegan), then that will be okay as the hero ingredients themselves haven't been removed. If you have an allergy to any hero ingredients, please omit them from the recipes.

A number of recipes in this book will call for legumes. Quantities used are from cans that have been drained and rinsed. If you want to reduce exposure to plastic from cans, you can simply substitute the approximate 400g of legumes with 100 grams of dried legumes and follow the cooking instructions on the packet.

## A Note on Cleaning Produce

Pesticides used on produce are known endocrine disruptors, which can cause hormone imbalances. Consuming organic products is best in reducing the chemicals in our bodies; however, this may not be possible. A way to remove pesticides is to soak them in vinegar or bi-carb soda for 15 minutes and then rinse. Studies have found that this process removes approximately 75 per cent of pesticide and 80 per cent of fungicide residue.

## A Final Note on the Power of Food

As you delve into the recipes and nutritional insights in the following chapters, remember that food is not merely sustenance; it's a powerful ally in fostering health, vitality and longevity. By aligning your dietary choices with the ebbs and flows of your menstrual cycle, you can embark on a journey of holistic wellbeing. Whether you have a natural cycle, are on hormonal birth control or face irregularities, these recipes are designed to cater to and support your unique nutritional needs.

So, let's embark on this culinary journey together, celebrating each phase of your cycle and embracing the profound connection between what you eat and how you feel. Nourishing your body appropriately is not just a good choice; it's a path to flourishing and living your healthiest, happiest life. Enjoy the recipes, embrace your cycle, and let the transformative power of food guide you toward a balanced and vibrant life.

# Pantry staples

The table below provides a list of pantry staples that feature regularly in many recipes. Having these on hand will make cooking according to your cycle much easier.

| | | | | |
|---|---|---|---|---|
| Nuts | Cashews<br>Almonds<br>Walnuts | | Oils | Olive oil<br>Coconut oil |
| Spices and seasoning | Cumin<br>Paprika<br>Coriander seeds<br>Oregano<br>Garlic powder<br>Cinnamon<br>Chilli powder<br>Cayenne pepper<br>Salt<br>Pepper | | Grains and seeds | Oats<br>Flaxseed meal<br>Buckwheat<br>Chia seeds<br>Pepitas<br>Sunflower seeds<br>Sesame seeds<br>(black and white)<br>Quinoa<br>Rice |
| Legumes | Lentils<br>Chickpeas<br>Red kidney beans<br>Black beans | | Other | Passata<br>Cacao powder<br>Smooth natural<br>nut butters*<br>Maple syrup<br>Coconut milk<br>Soy sauce/tamari<br>Vinegars<br>Canned tomatoes<br>Tomato paste<br>Vegetable stock |

* Make sure whatever you choose is natural and smooth, as the texture and taste will change if using other products.

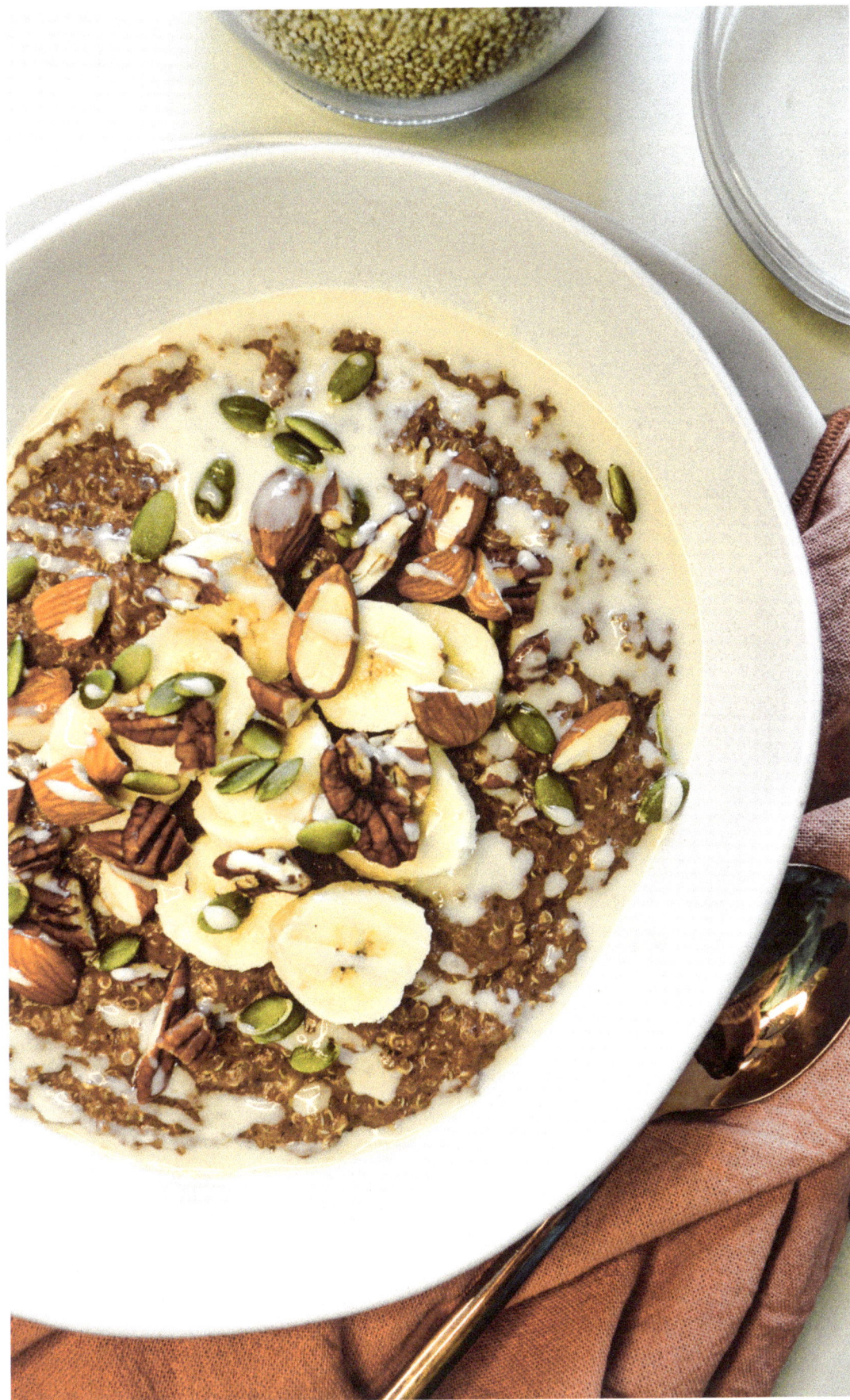

menstrual phase

# HERO FOODS

## NUTRIENTS FOR THE MENSTRUAL PHASE

IRON | ZINC | MAGNESIUM | VITAMIN C

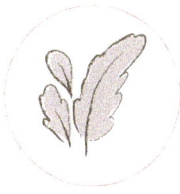

LEAFY GREENS

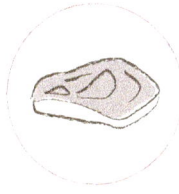

BEEF & DUCK

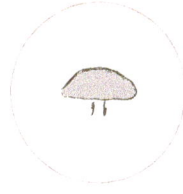

MUSHROOMS

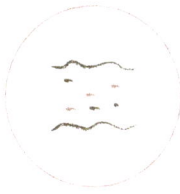

NORI

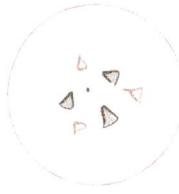

BUCKWHEAT

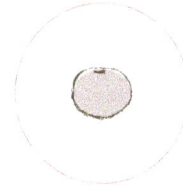

BLUEBERRIES

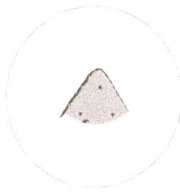

MISO

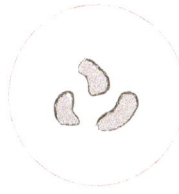

BEANS

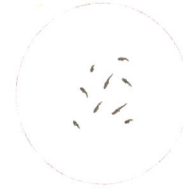

WILD RICE

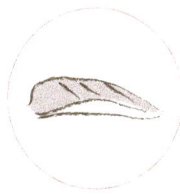

FISH
(FATTY & SHELL)

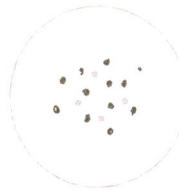

LENTILS

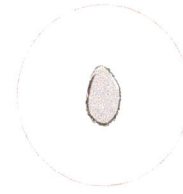

EGGS

# menstrual recipes

# breakfast

Rest & Replenish
Smoothie

Speedy
Spicy Beans

Wild Mushroom,
Wilted Spinach &
Polenta

Buckwheat
Pancake Bowls

Baked Egg &
Mushroom Cups

Steak & Eggs
with Balsamic Mushrooms
and Rocket Pesto

Buckwheat Porridge
with Berry Compote

# REST & REPLENISH SMOOTHIE

**Serves:** 1    **Prep:** 5 minutes    **Cook:** N/A

1 cup beetroot, peeled and diced
1 tsp cacao powder
½ cup frozen blueberries or blackberries
1 cup spinach or kale
1 tbsp almond butter
1 tbsp sunflower seeds
1 tbsp chia seeds
1 cup warm water
½ tsp cinnamon
1 heaped tablespoon protein powder

Add all the ingredients into a blender and blend until smooth. Serve immediately.

*This recipe also doubles as a snack option.*

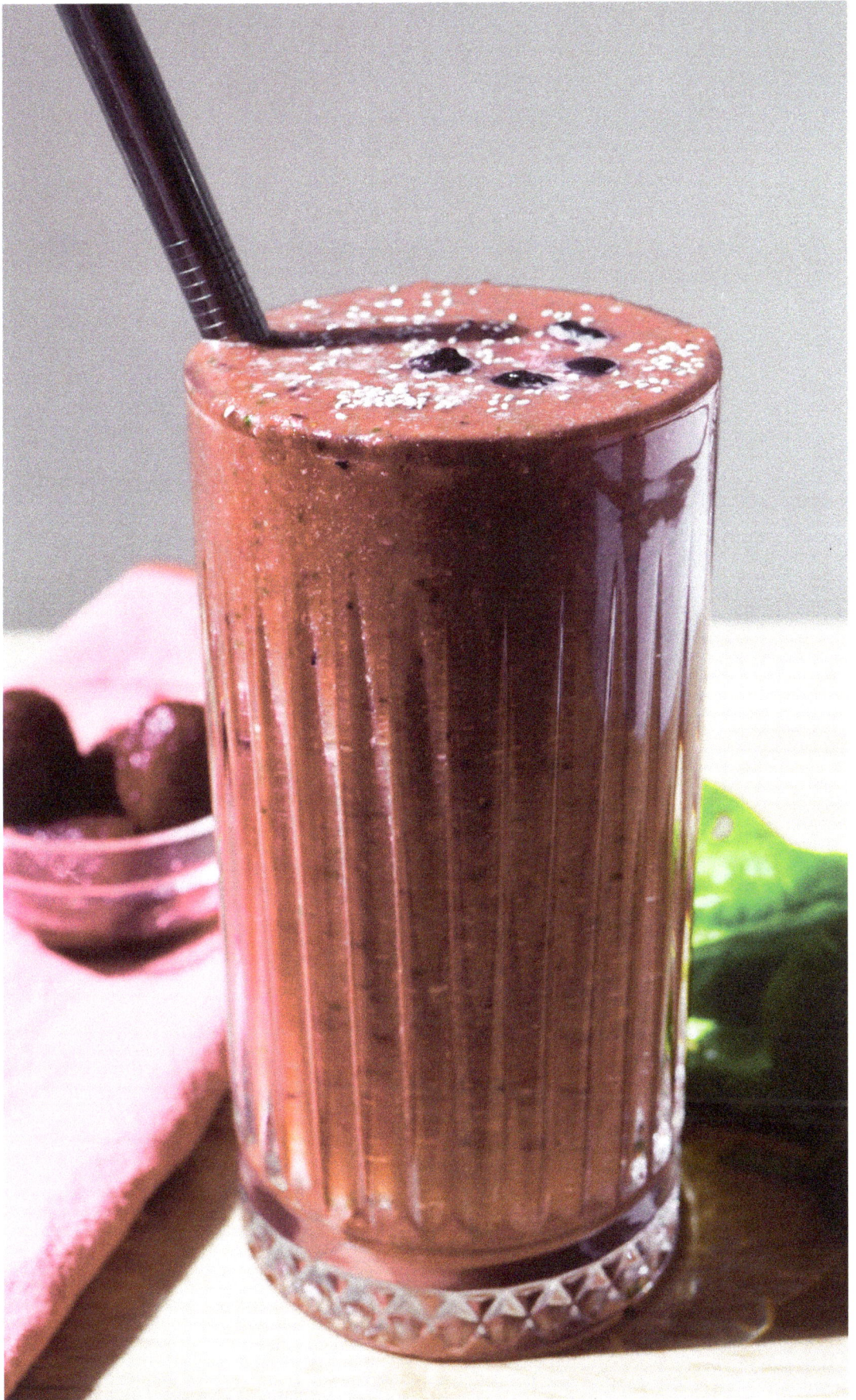

# SPEEDY SPICY BEANS

**Serves:** 4     **Prep:** 5 minutes     **Cook:** 20 minutes

1 tbsp olive oil
1 onion, diced
2 garlic cloves, minced
2 tbsp dried oregano
1 tsp chilli flakes (adjust to
  your preference)
4 tbsp tomato paste
700g passata
⅓ cup red wine vinegar
3 cups water
2 bay leaves
400g can mixed beans,
  drained
400g can white beans,
  drained
1 cup dried green lentils*

**To serve:**
Poached eggs (1-2 per
  serve)
Sourdough bread
Hemp seeds (optional,
  1 tbsp per serve)
Parsley, chopped (optional)

Heat a pot on medium with oil and add the onion and garlic. Cook for a few minutes until softened.

Add the oregano, chilli flakes and tomato paste to the pan. Stir to combine.

Add the passata, red wine vinegar, water, bay leaves, beans and lentils. Cook for about 25-30 minutes, until the lentils have softenen and the sauce has thickened. Season with salt and pepper to taste.

Serve over sourdough bread, poached eggs and sprinkle with hemp seeds and parsley.

**NOTE:**
› To reduce cooking time, you can use 400g of canned lentils (drain and rinse them, and reduce the water to 1 cup). Alternatively, use pre-soaked dried lentils and reduce the cooking time by about 10-15 minutes.

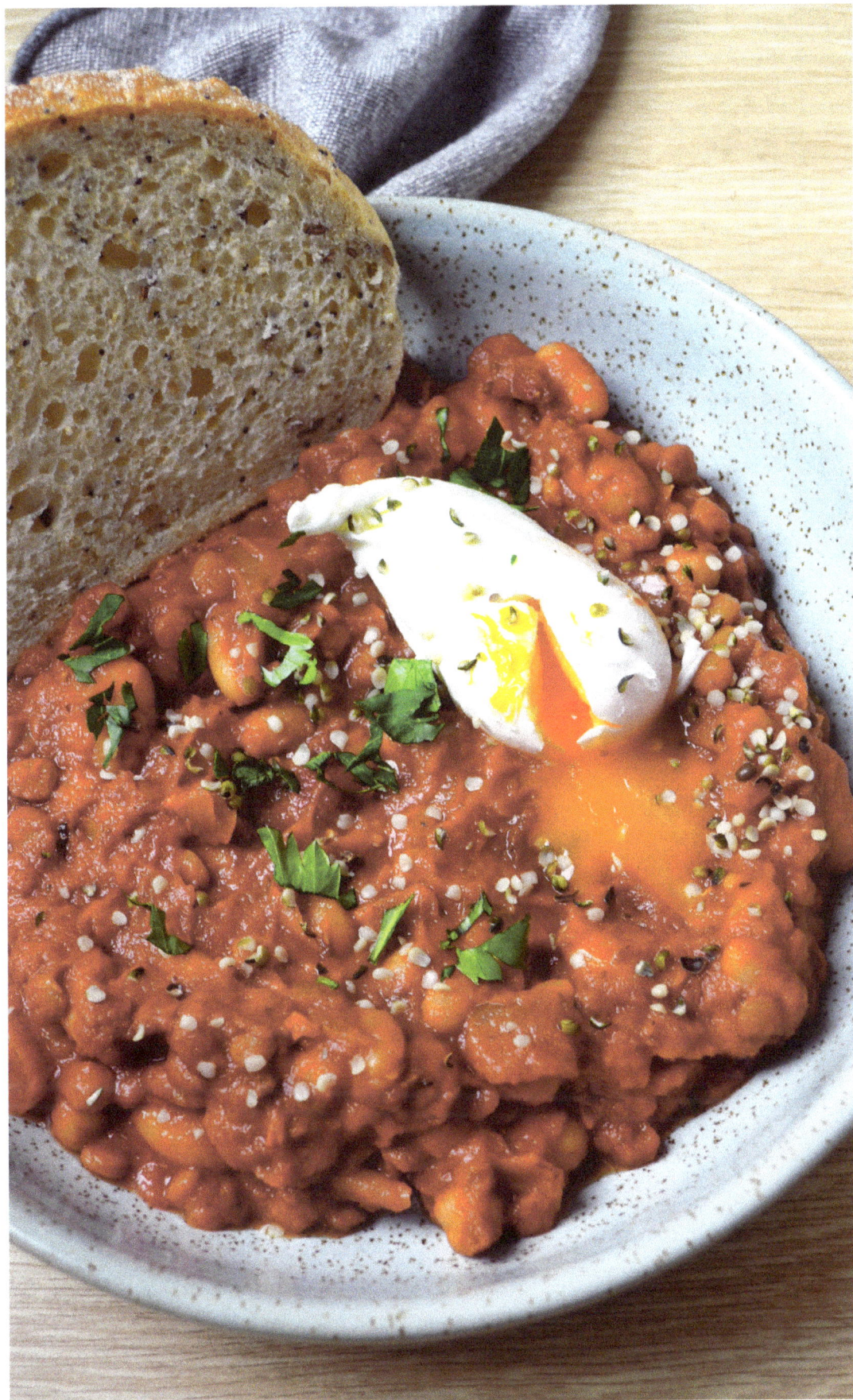

# WILD MUSHROOM, WILTED SPINACH & POLENTA

**Serves:** 4    **Prep:** 10 minutes    **Cook:** 30 minutes

5 cups bone broth (see page 245)
1 cup polenta
1 cup water
1 tsp butter
Salt and pepper to season
1 tsp olive oil
4 brown mushrooms
4 white mushrooms
320g enoki mushrooms
4 garlic cloves, crushed
1 tbsp dried thyme
2 cups spinach, roughly chopped

**To serve:**
Poached eggs
Goat cheese, crumbled
Parsley, chopped

In a saucepan on medium heat, bring the bone broth to a boil. Reduce to a simmer on a low heat and slowly pour in the polenta while stirring with your other hand. Stir continuously for about 5 minutes. Add half the water and cover with a lid for about 20 minutes, stirring every couple minutes to avoid the polenta sticking to the pan. Once the polenta thickens and becomes creamy and firm, add the remaining water and stir through. Add the butter and season with salt and pepper.

While the polenta is cooking, heat a pan on medium–low heat. Add the olive oil and all the mushrooms, sautéing for 5 minutes. Add the garlic and thyme and continue to cook for another 2 minutes. Add the spinach and cook until the spinach has wilted.

In a bowl, add the polenta and mushrooms. Top with a poached egg, crumbled goat cheese and parsley.

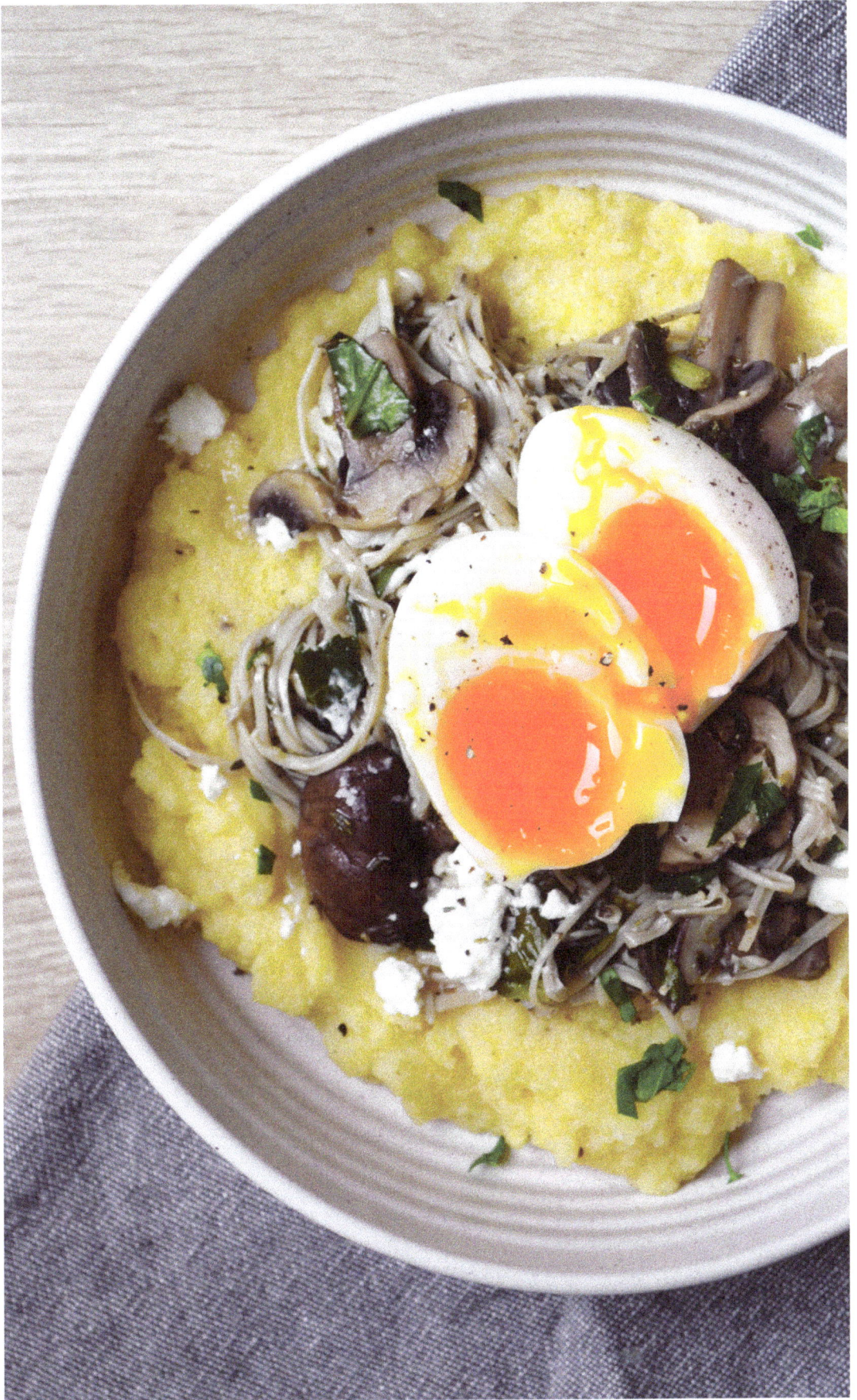

# BUCKWHEAT PANCAKE BOWLS

**Serves:** 2     **Prep:** 5 minutes     **Cook:** 30 minutes

**For the pancakes:**
½ cup buckwheat groats
1 tbsp vanilla protein
   powder
2 tbsp chia seeds
300g ricotta
1 lemon, juiced and zested
2 eggs
⅓ cup milk (of choice)
½ tsp baking powder
1 tsp vanilla essence
½ cup blueberries

**For the whipped ricotta:**
125g ricotta
2 tsp honey

**Optional toppings:**
Blueberries or berry
   compote (see page 145)
Lemon zest
Sunflower seeds

Preheat the oven to 180°C fan-forced.

In a blender, add the buckwheat groats and blend until a flour-like texture forms. Add the protein powder, chia seeds, ricotta, lemon juice and zest, eggs, milk, baking powder and vanilla essence and blend until smooth. Transfer the mixture to two single-serve glass baking dishes and stir through the blueberries. Bake in the oven for 25–30 minutes or until the mixture is firm.

Make the whipped ricotta by adding the ricotta and honey to a blender and blend for 1–2 minutes until smooth and creamy.

Serve the baked pancake with the whipped ricotta and top with extra blueberries or berry compote, lemon zest and sunflower seeds if desired.

**TIP:**
› Use buckwheat groats and mill them in a food processor to make your own flour.

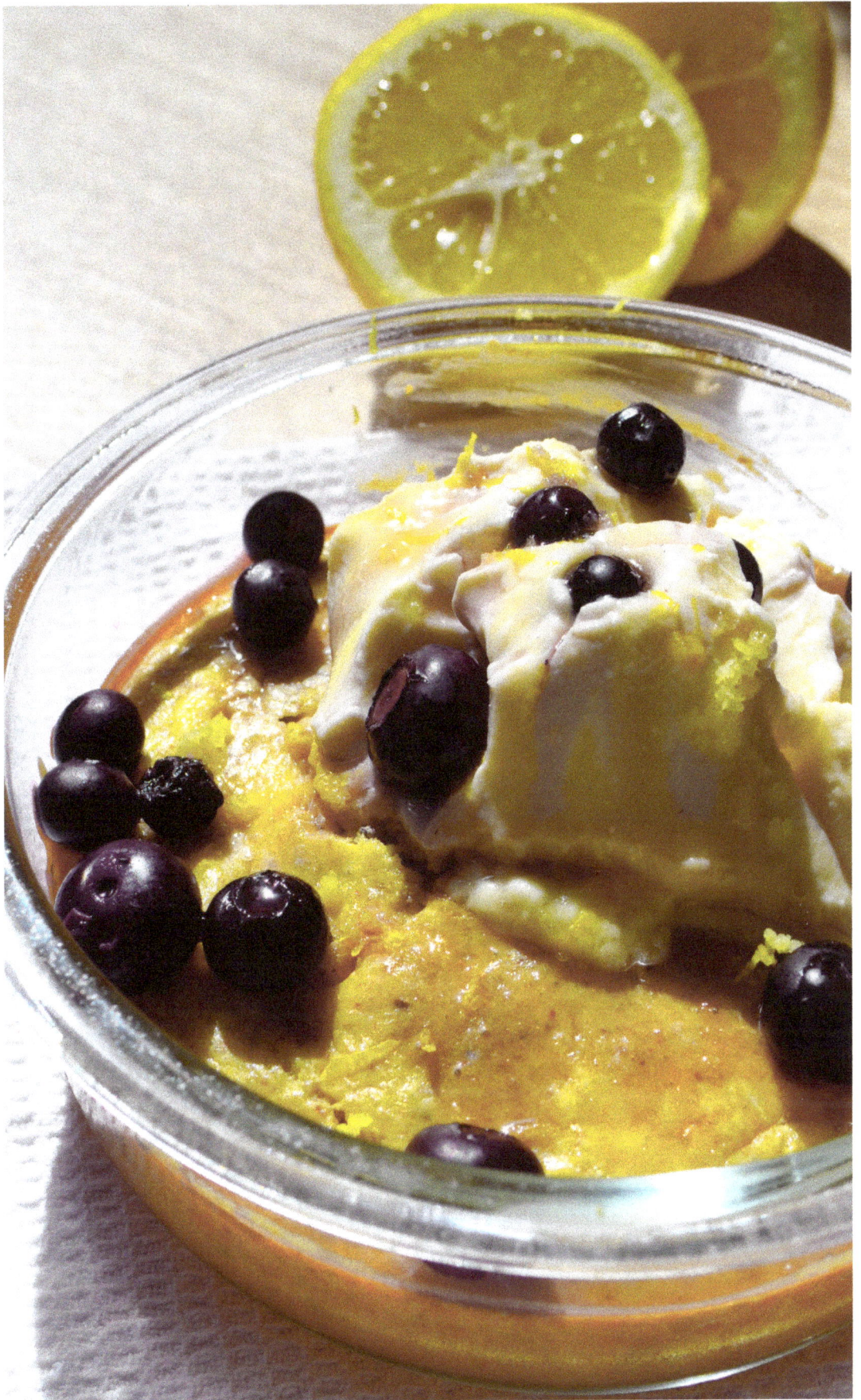

# BAKED EGG & MUSHROOM CUPS

**Serves:** 4     **Prep:** 5 minutes     **Cook:** 30–40 minutes

Olive oil/butter
4 large flat mushrooms
4 fresh thyme sprigs, leaves
  plucked
1 garlic clove, grated
Salt and pepper
4 eggs
4 tomatoes, halved

To serve:
Rocket
Avocado
Sourdough bread

Preheat the oven to 180°C fan-forced.

Grease ramekins with olive oil or butter then place the mushrooms in the ramekins. Season the mushroom with the thyme leaves, grated garlic, salt and pepper. Bake in the oven for 10 minutes.

Remove the mushrooms from the oven and crack an egg into each one. Return the mushrooms to the oven and cook for another 10–15 minutes, until the eggs are cooked to your liking.

In a separate baking dish, add the halved tomatoes and season with salt and pepper. Bake for 10-15 minutes.

Serve the mushroom, eggs and tomato with rocket, avocado and sourdough bread for a complete meal.

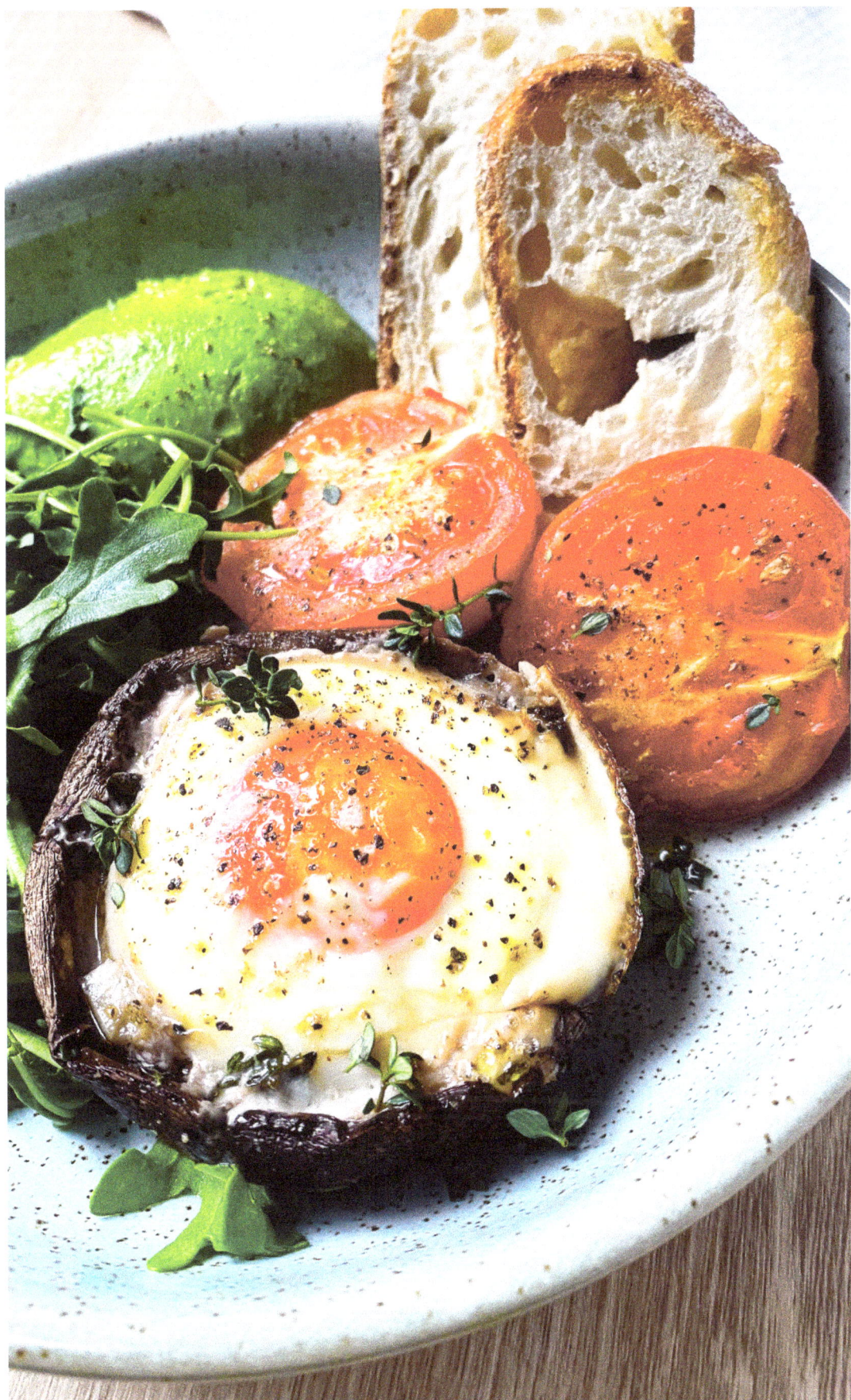

# STEAK & EGGS
## WITH BALSAMIC MUSHROOMS AND ROCKET PESTO

**Serves:** 2    **Prep:** 5 minutes    **Cook:** 20 minutes

4-6 pieces of beef sizzle
  steak
Salt and pepper
½ tsp olive oil
1 small brown onion, sliced
  (optional)
6 button mushrooms, sliced
1 tbsp balsamic vinegar
2 tomatoes, halved
2 eggs
½ cup rocket

For the rocket pesto:
1 cup rocket
1 garlic clove
2 tbsp olive oil
Salt and pepper

Optional sides:
Avocado
Sourdough bread

To make the pesto, add the rocket, garlic, olive oil and a pinch of salt and pepper to a food processor. Blend until well combined. Set aside.

Season the steaks with salt and pepper. Heat a pan on medium with ½ teaspoon of olive oil. Add the sizzle steaks and cook for 1 minute per side. Remove from pan and allow to rest.

Add the onions to the same pan and sauté for 2 minutes. Then add the mushrooms and balsamic vinegar and cook for another 2 minutes. Add the tomatoes and cook until soft.

Cook the eggs to your preference: boiled, poached, sunny side up or scrambled.

Serve the steaks, eggs, tomatoes and mushrooms and top with the rocket pesto and extra rocket on the side. If desired, serve with avocado and sourdough bread.

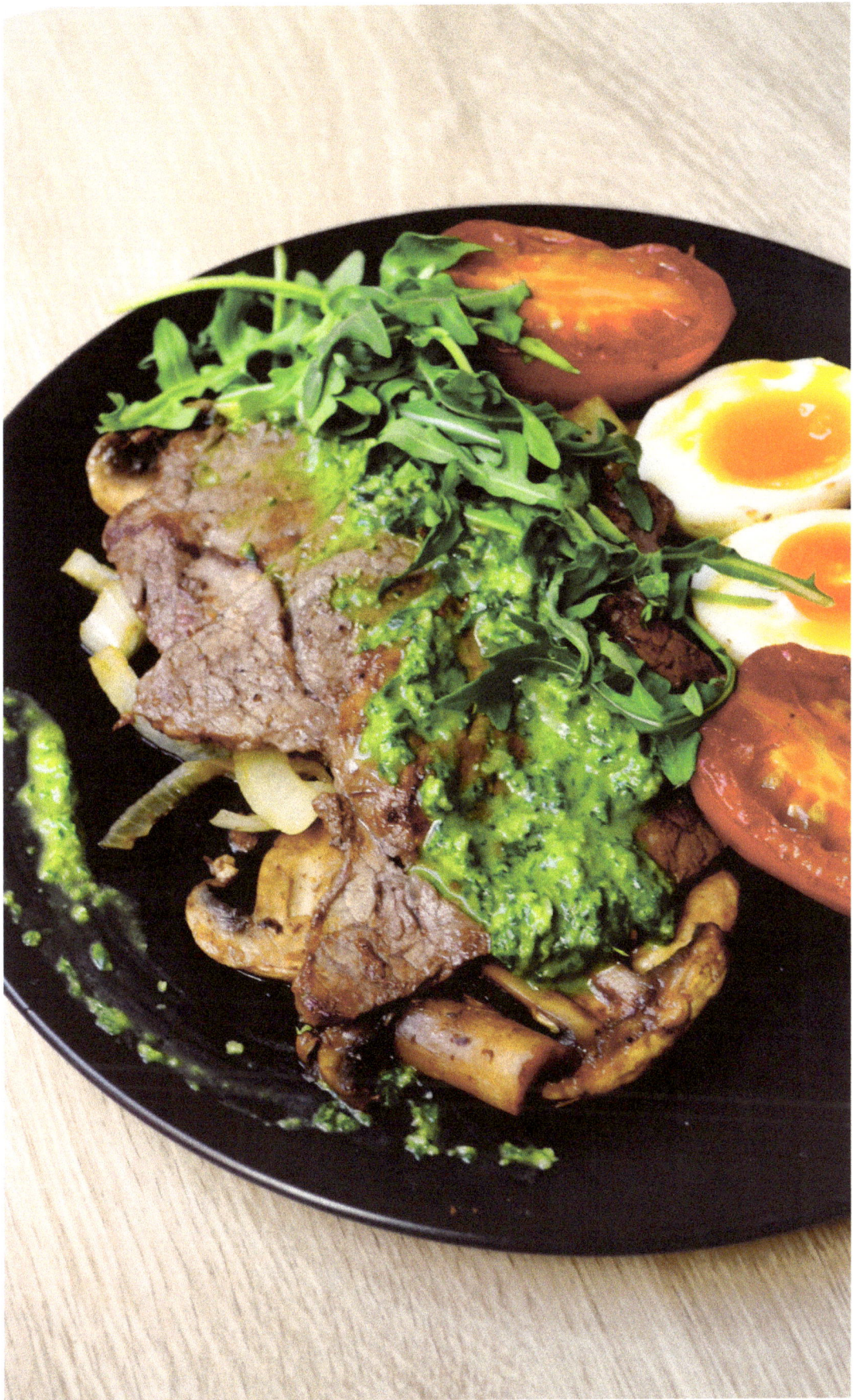

# BUCKWHEAT PORRIDGE
## WITH BERRY COMPOTE

**Serves:** 2     **Prep:** 25 minutes     **Cook:** 20 minutes

1 ½ cups raw buckwheat groats
¼ cup sunflower seeds
2 cups water
2 cups unsweetened almond milk
2 tbsp chia seeds
2 heaped tbsp vanilla or plain protein powder
2 tbsp almond butter
1 tsp cinnamon
1 tsp raw cacao powder (optional)

**For the berry compote:**
1 cup blueberries
½ tbsp lemon juice
¼ cup water

**Optional toppings:**
Greek yoghurt
Banana
Honey or maple syrup
Sunflower seeds
Raw buckwheat groats

Soak the buckwheat groats in water and set aside for 20 minutes.

Drain the buckwheat and then combine it with the sunflower seeds, water and almond milk in a pot.

Cover and bring to a boil over medium heat, stirring occasionally. When boiled, reduce to a simmer uncovered. Add the chia seeds and protein powder and stir through. Cook for 10 minutes, stirring frequently, until the buckwheat is tender and creamy.

Stir through the almond butter, cinnamon and cacao (if using). If desired, use a stick blender to make it even more smooth and creamy. Ensure that you leave some liquid as this will thicken when cooled. If needed, add more milk or water.

To make the berry compote, add the berries, lemon juice and water to a small pot. Bring to a simmer and reduce. Cook until the berries are soft enough to mash.

Serve the porridge in a bowl and top with the berry compote. Serve with banana, Greek yoghurt, extra sunflower seeds or raw buckwheat groats, maple syrup or honey.

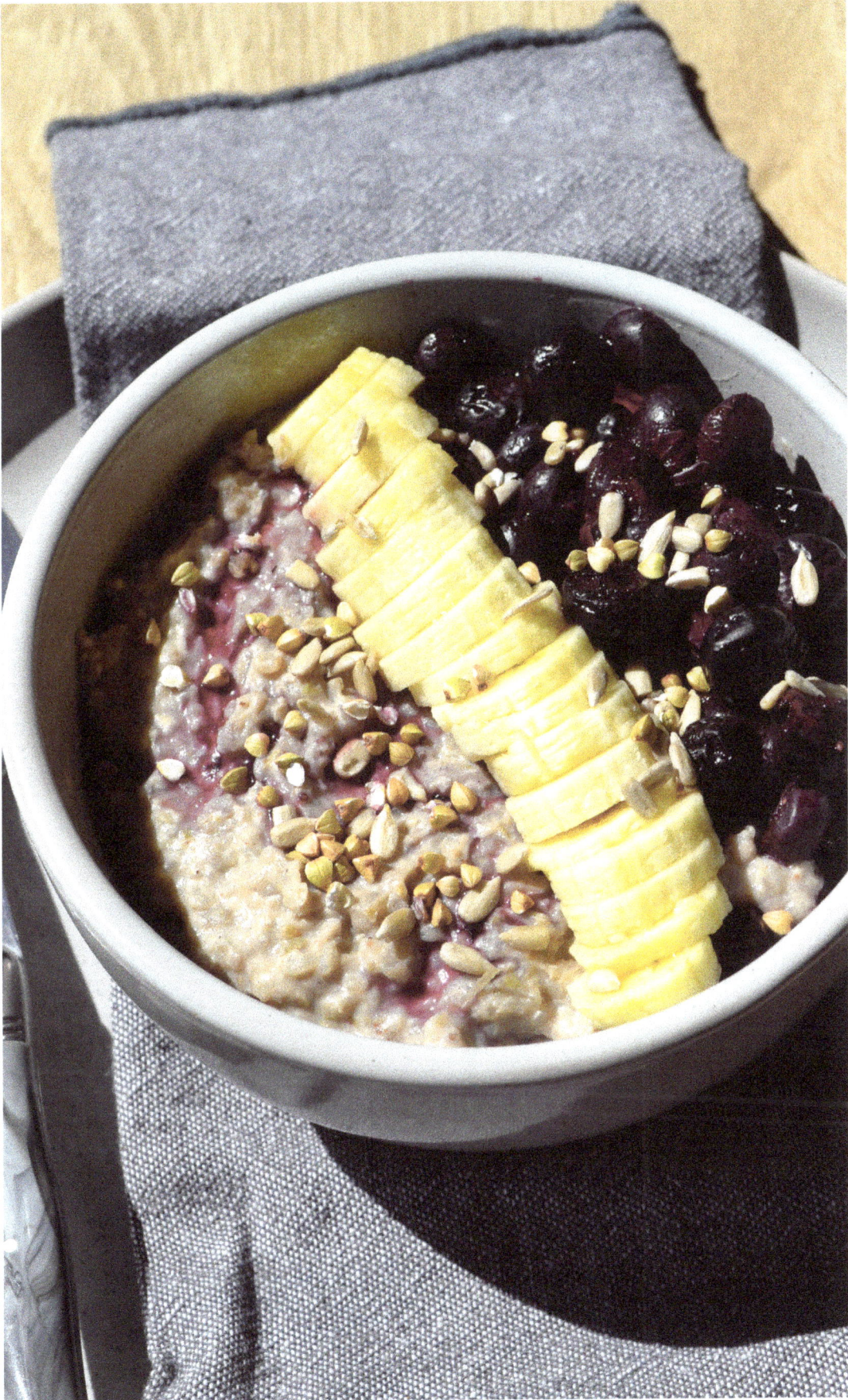

# mains

Salmon
Nourish Bowls

Beets & Beans

Mushroom
Stroganoff

Mushroom Chilli

Beef Stirfry

Beef Fajitas

Beef Pho

Taco Soup

Duck &
Miso Soup

Prawn Red Curry

# SALMON NOURISH BOWLS

**Serves:** 2     **Prep:** 5 minutes     **Cook:** 20 minutes

2 tsp miso paste
1 tbsp Dijon mustard
1 tbsp rice wine vinegar
1 tsp soy sauce/tamari
1 tsp honey
1 tsp olive oil
2 salmon fillets
4 mushrooms, quartered
1 head broccoli, cut into
  florets

Sushi seasoning:
1 packet (5g) seaweed
  snack, finely chopped
1 tbsp black sesame seeds
1 tbsp white sesame seeds
1 tsp sea salt

To serve:
2 cups wild rice, cooked
1 avocado, halved and
  sliced
1 cucumber, sliced

Preheat the oven to 180°C fan-forced.

In a bowl, combine the miso paste, Dijon mustard, rice wine vinegar, soy sauce/tamari, honey and olive oil and stir. Add the salmon fillets and mushrooms to the bowl and coat the marinade evenly over them.

On a lined baking tray, add the broccoli and drizzle with olive oil. Add the salmon and mushrooms to the tray and bake in the oven for 15–20 minutes.

Meanwhile, make the sushi seasoning by combining the chopped seaweed snack, sesame seeds and salt in a jar. Set aside.

Serve the salmon and broccoli on a bed of wild rice, with sliced avocado and pickled cucumbers. Top with sushi seasoning.

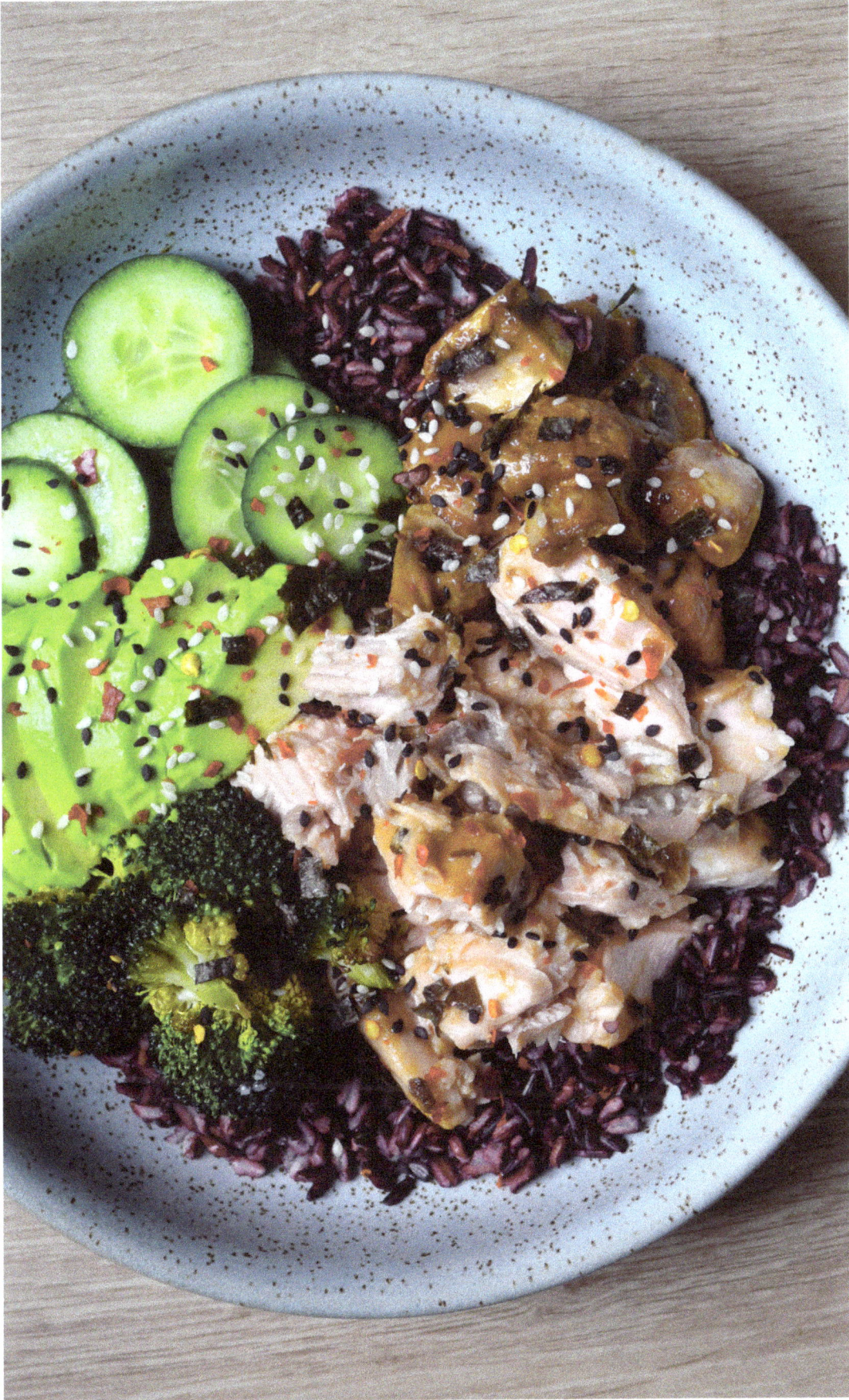

# BEETS & BEANS

**Serves:** 3-4      **Prep:** 10 minutes      **Cook:** 30 minutes

3 large beetroots, peeled
  and diced
3 cups water
1 cup dried red lentils
170g Greek yoghurt
2 tbsp dried dill
1 lemon, juiced
2 garlic cloves
Salt and pepper
1 tsp olive oil
800g butterbeans, rinsed
  and drained

To serve:
100g feta
¼ cup walnuts, roughly
  chopped
¼ cup sunflower seeds
¼ cup hemp seeds
Fresh mint or dill (optional)
Sourdough bread, toasted
  (optional)

Half fill a pot with water and bring to the boil before placing a steaming basket on top. Add the diced beetroot to the steaming basket, cover with a lid and steam for 20 minutes until the beetroot is tender.

In another pot, add 3 cups of water and the dried red lentils. Bring to the boil and simmer for 10 minutes or until tender, stirring regularly.

Then in a food processor add the steamed beetroot, lentils, Greek yoghurt, dill, lemon juice, garlic and salt and pepper. Blend until well combined and smooth.

Heat a pan on low-medium heat. Add the olive oil and butterbeans. Sauté the beans for 3 minutes. Pour in the beetroot mix and stir through, cooking for 5 minutes.

Serve into 3-4 dishes and add the toppings, evenly dividing the feta, walnuts, sunflower seeds, hemp seeds, fresh herbs and toasted sourdough bread, if desired.

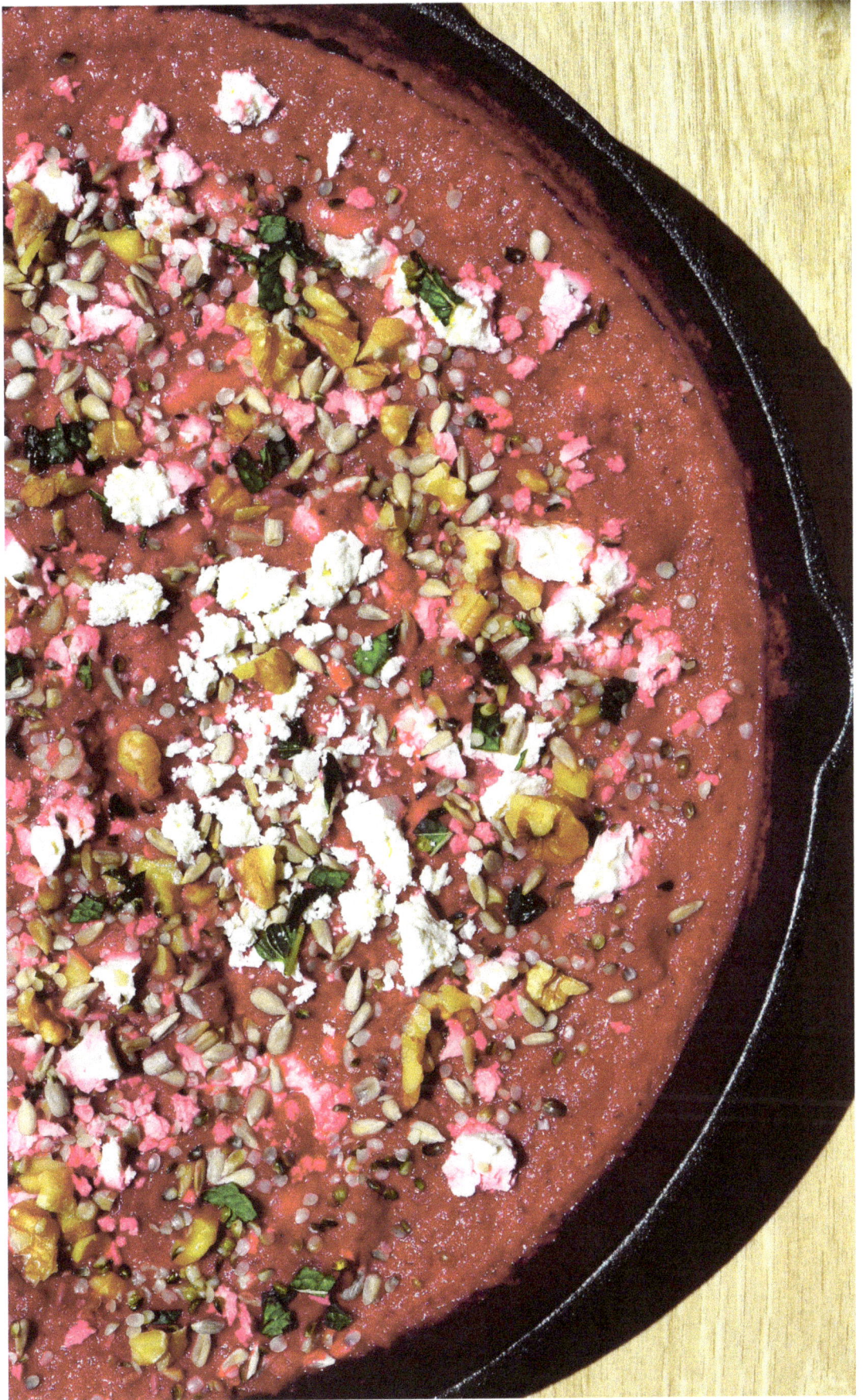

# MUSHROOM STROGANOFF

**Serves:** 4    **Prep:** 10 minutes    **Cook:** 15 minutes

Olive oil
2 garlic cloves, crushed
1 white onion
½ bunch parsley leaves and
  stems, chopped
500g mushrooms, sliced
1 tbsp sweet paprika
1 tbsp dried or fresh thyme
1 tbsp soy sauce/tamari
3 tbsp worcestershire sauce
2 tbsp nutritional yeast
2 tsp Dijon mustard
400ml canned coconut
  milk
3 cups spinach
2 cups wild/black rice,
  cooked

In a large pan on medium heat, add a drizzle of olive oil and sauté the garlic, onion and chopped parsley stems for 2-3 minutes.

Add the mushrooms in batches, cooking down for about 5 minutes. Add the paprika, thyme, soy sauce/tamari, worcestershire sauce, nutritional yeast, Dijon and coconut milk. Simmer for 5 minutes.

Add the spinach and parsley leaves and allow to wilt. Season with salt and pepper.

Serve with wild rice and garnish with parsley if desired.

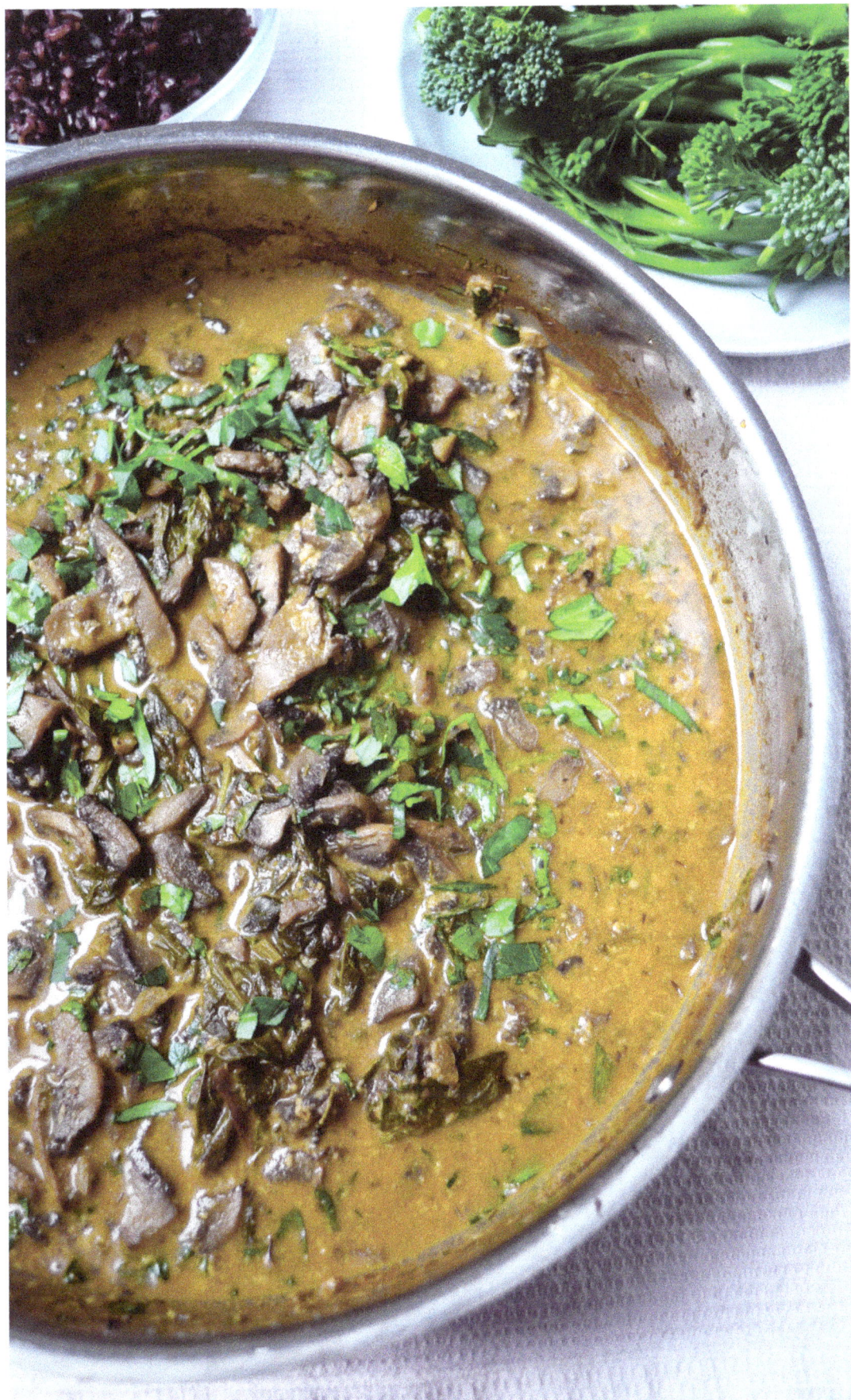

# MUSHROOM CHILLI

**Serves:** 4      **Prep:** 15 minutes      **Cook:** 20 minutes

1 brown onion, quartered
1 garlic clove, chopped
1 tbsp olive oil
8 mushrooms
1 green capsicum, diced
1 jalapeno (or 5 pickled
  jalapeno pieces), chopped
1 ½ tsp dried oregano
¼ tsp chilli powder
  (adjusted to taste)
1 tsp ground cumin
½ tsp paprika
400g diced tomatoes
400g canned kidney beans,
  drained and rinsed
Salt and pepper

**To serve:**
Avocado
Spinach, chopped
Quinoa and brown rice
Coriander
Pico de gallo (optional)

In a food processor, add the onion and garlic to finely chop. Heat a frypan to medium heat with the olive oil and sauté the onion and garlic for a couple of minutes.

Meanwhile, add the mushrooms to the food processor and chop until a mince-like texture has formed. Add the mushrooms to the pan and sauté for a few minutes.

Add the capsicum and jalapeno to the pan along with the oregano, chilli powder, cumin and paprika. Cook for a further 5 minutes or until the capsicum has softened slightly.

Add the diced tomatoes and beans to the pan and bring to a simmer, allowing the sauce to thicken. Season with salt and pepper as desired.

Serve with toppings and sides of choice.

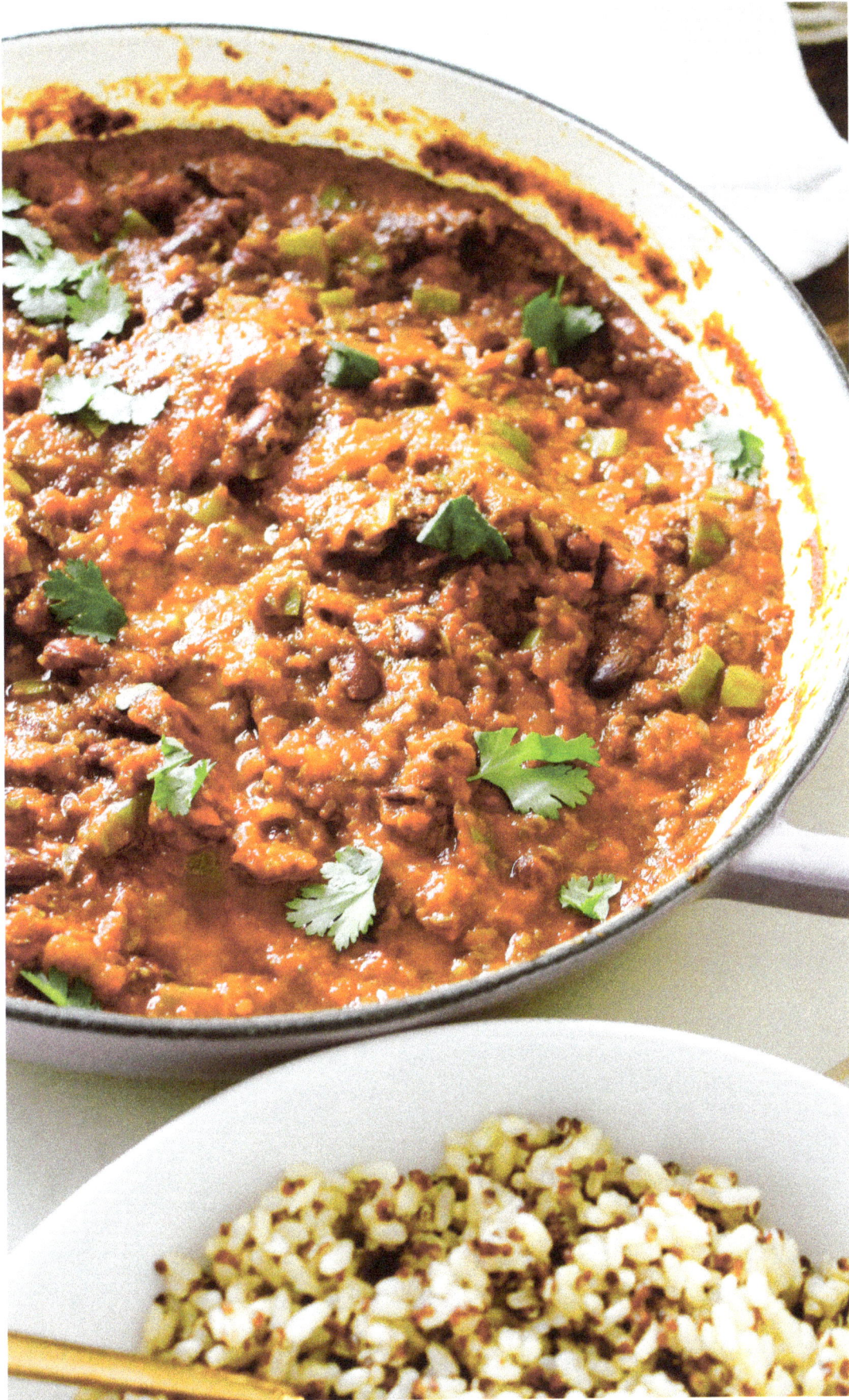

# BEEF STIRFRY

**Serves:** 4      **Prep:** 10 minutes      **Cook:** 20 minutes

1 tsp olive oil
1 red onion, finely sliced
2 garlic cloves, grated
1 tbsp grated ginger
1 bunch Chinese broccoli
500g beef mince
2 tbsp tamari/soy sauce
1 tsp Chinese five spice
1 tbsp water
1 red capsicum, finely sliced
1 bunch broccolini, chopped
225g water chestnuts,
   drained, rinsed and
   chopped

**For the sweet chilli sauce
(optional):**
2 tbsp honey
1 tbsp rice wine vinegar
1 tsp chilli flakes (adjusted
   to taste)
1 lime, zested and juiced
1 tsp tamari/soy sauce
1 tsp ginger, grated
1 garlic, grated

**To serve:**
Noodles or rice of choice
   (Soba noodles are
   preferred for the
   Menstrual Phase)
Sesame seeds
Lime
Coriander, mint and/or
   Thai basil (optional)
Spring onions, sliced
   (optional)

In a pan on medium heat, warm the olive oil and then add the red onion, garlic, ginger and Chinese broccoli, sautéing for a few minutes until the onions have slightly softened and the broccoli has slightly wilted. Remove just the broccoli and set aside, covering to keep warm. Then add the beef mince and cook for 5–7 minutes until cooked through. Stir through the tamari/soy sauce, Chinese five spice and water and cook for another 5 minutes.

Add the capsicum, broccolini and water chestnuts and cook through for 5 minutes until tender.

Meanwhile, make the sweet chilli sauce by combining the honey, rice wine vinegar, chilli flakes (adjusted to taste), lime zest and juice, tamari/soy sauce, ginger and garlic in a small bowl.

When ready to serve, add the beef stir fry and Chinese broccoli to bowls with the noodles or rice of choice. Garnish with herbs, spring onions and sesame seeds if desired. Finish by drizzling the sweet chilli sauce over the stir fry.

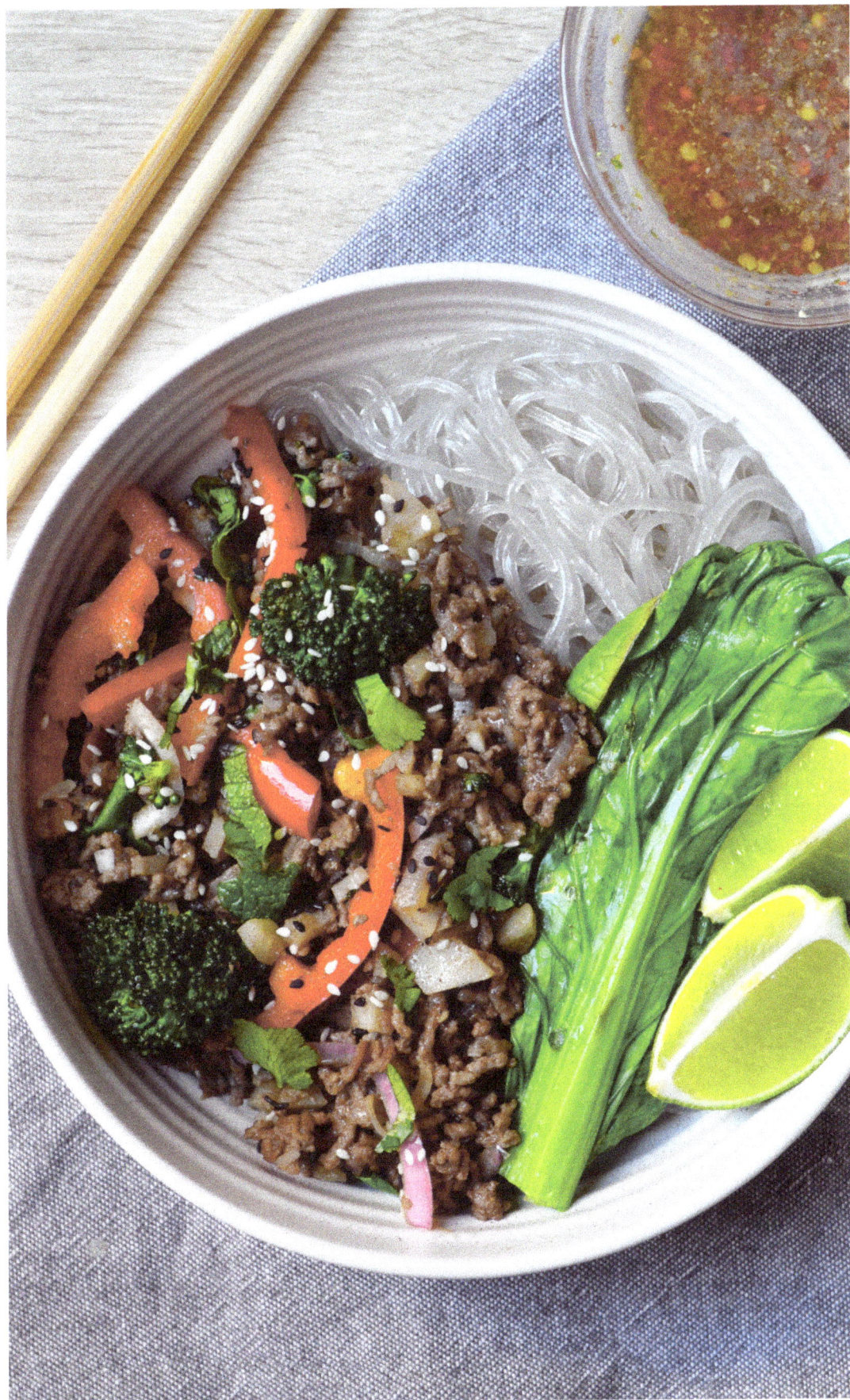

# BEEF FAJITAS

**Serves:** 4      **Prep:** 10 minutes      **Cook:** 10 minutes

1 tsp olive oil
500g beef strips
1 white onion, sliced
1 red onion, sliced
3 capsicums (red, yellow
  and green), sliced
400g canned kidney beans,
  drained and rinsed
1 tsp cumin
1 tsp paprika
1 tsp oregano
½ tsp garlic powder
2 tbsp water

**To serve:**
Tortilla wraps of choice
Guacamole
Lime wedge

In a fry pan on medium heat, add the oil and the beef strips, in batches, and cook for 2 minutes. Remove from the pan.

Add the onions and capsicum to the pan and sauté for 5 minutes. Add the kidney beans, spices and water and continue cooking for a further 5 minutes.

Return the beef to the pan and stir through.

Serve the fajita mix with tortilla wraps and guacamole.

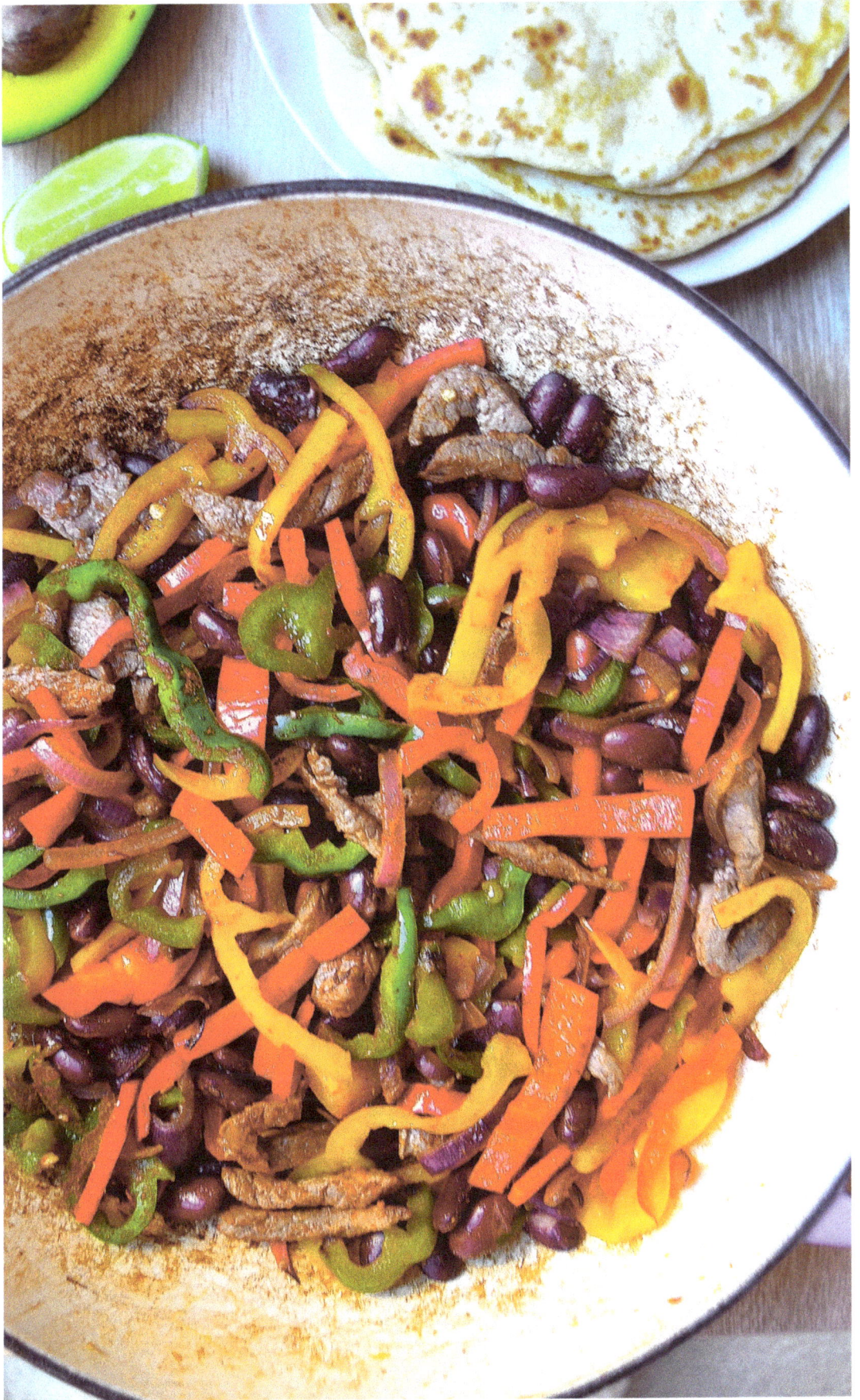

# BEEF PHO

**Serves:** 4     **Prep:** 10 minutes     **Cook:** 15 minutes

500g oyster blade steaks
4 cups bone broth (for homemade, see page 245)
2 cups water
1 ½ tsp ground Chinese five spice
2 tbsp ginger, grated
3 garlic cloves, grated
½ red chilli, sliced (optional)
1 tbsp fish sauce
1 tbsp lime juice
140g soba noodles
6 shitake mushrooms, sliced
1 bunch Chinese broccoli, chopped
2 bunches bok choy, sliced
Salt and pepper to taste

To garnish:
2 cups bean shoots
Coriander leaves (optional)
½ red chilli, sliced
Lime wedge (optional)

Place the oyster blade steaks on a plate and put in the freezer. This will make it easier to thinly slice the beef when serving.

In a large pot on medium heat, add your bone broth and water. Then add the Chinese five spice, ginger, garlic, chilli, fish sauce and lime juice. Bring to a boil and reduce to a simmer.

In a glass bowl, cook the noodles by covering them with some of the bone broth and leaving for 5 minutes.

Add the shitake mushrooms to the broth in the pot. Once the noodles have cooked, add the chinese broccoli and bok choy to the pot. Turn off the heat and allow them to lightly wilt.

Remove the beef from the freezer and slice thinly.

To serve, divide the noodles between the bowls then top with the sliced beef. Pour over the hot broth - this will cook the beef to about medium rare (if you want your beef to be cooked completely, just allow it to sit in the broth for longer). Top with bean sprouts, coriander, sliced chilli and a lime wedge, if desired.

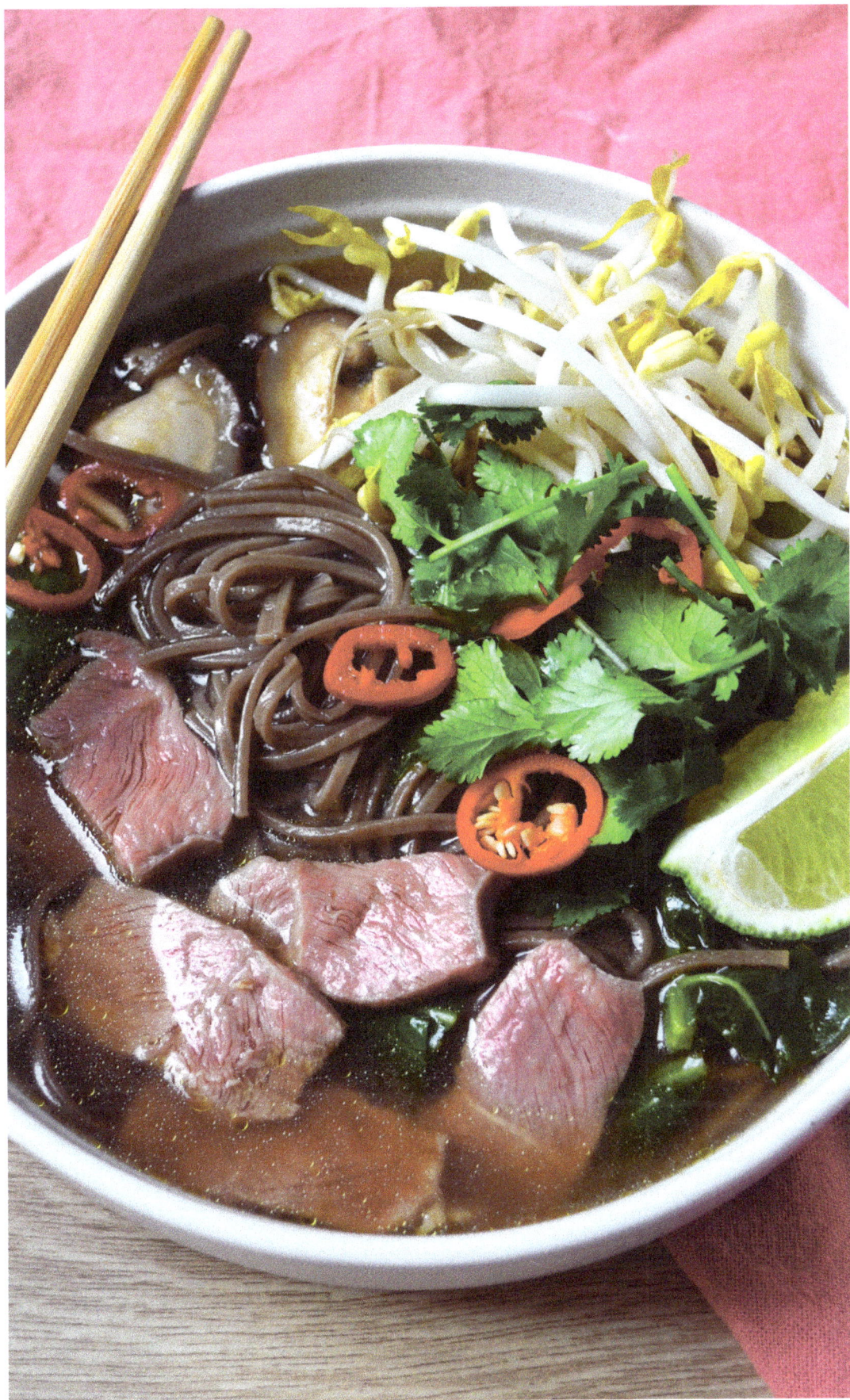

# TACO SOUP

**Serves:** 4    **Prep:** 10 minutes    **Cook:** 3.5 hours

**For the slow-cooked beef:**
500g chuck steak
Pinch of salt and pepper
Olive oil
1 onion, diced
1 garlic clove, chopped
4 cups beef stock or bone
  broth (see page 245)
1 tsp salt

**For the soup base:**
400g canned diced
  tomatoes
400g canned black beans,
  drained and rinsed
400g canned mixed beans,
  drained and rinsed
1 red capsicum, diced
400g canned corn kernels,
  drained
1 tbsp cumin
1 tbsp paprika
1 tbsp oregano
½ tbsp garlic power
Pinch of salt and pepper

**To serve:**
Toasted tortilla pieces
Coriander leaves
Avocado, diced

Season the steak with a pinch of salt and pepper. Heat a casserole dish on medium with a drizzle of olive oil and add the beef, browning for about 1 minute on each side. Set aside.

In the same pot or in a slow cooker, add the onion and garlic and sauté for 2-3 minutes until soft. Return the beef to the pot and add the stock and salt. Cover with a lid and simmer on a low heat for 3 hours.

Once cooked, remove the beef from the pot and shred using two forks. Return to pot and add the diced tomatoes, beans, capsicum, corn, cumin, paprika, oregano and garlic powder. Season with salt and pepper as desired. Simmer on a low heat for 15 minutes.

Serve with toasted tortilla pieces, coriander, cheese, avocado and a squeeze of lime juice.

**NOTES:**
› To save time on this dish, purchase pre-prepared slow-cooked pulled beef or use shredded roast chicken as an alternative to beef.
› **Make it plant based:** Replace the beef stock with vegetable stock and the chuck steak with additional beans.

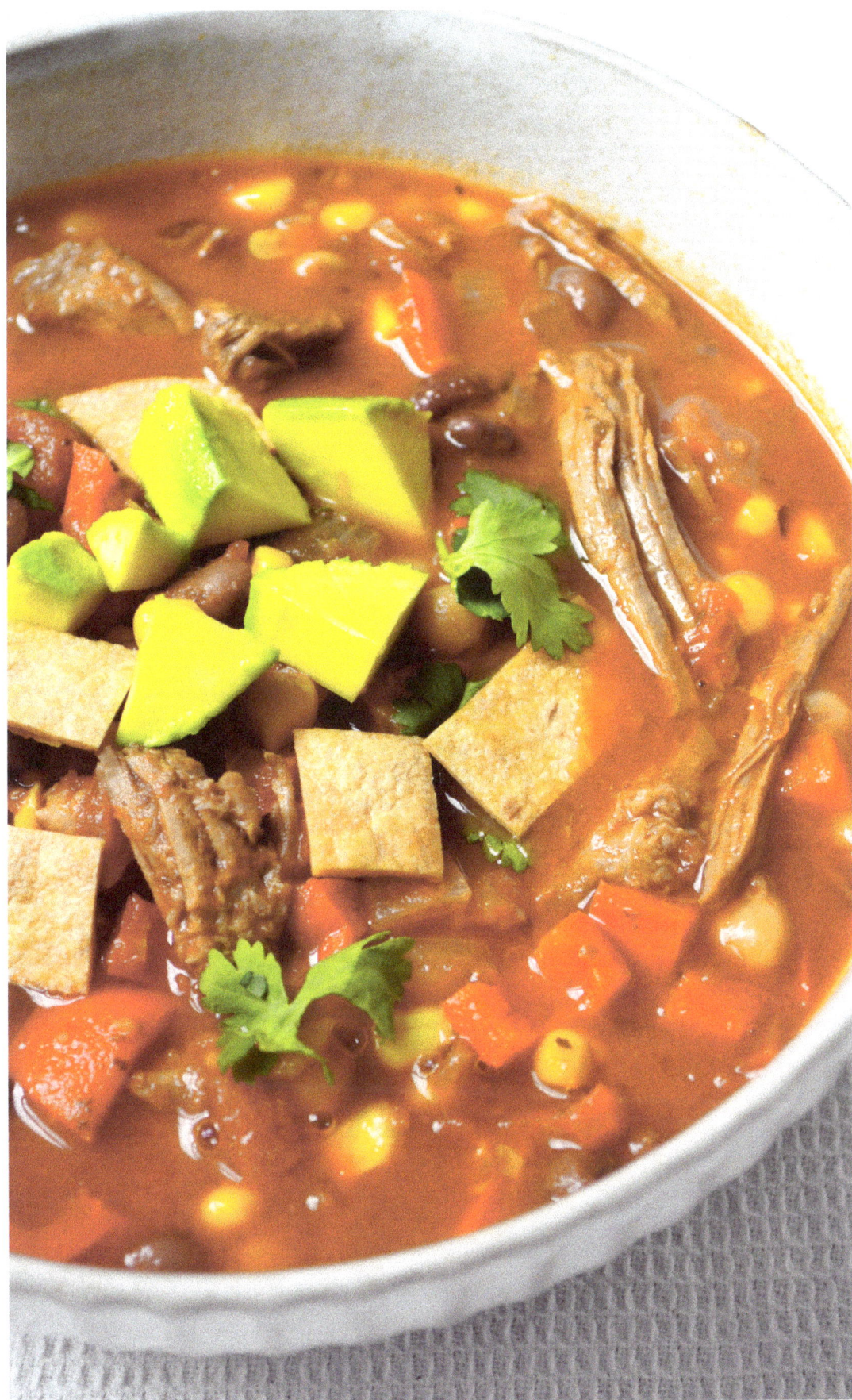

# DUCK & MISO SOUP

**Serves:** 2     **Prep:** 10 minutes     **Cook:** 20 minutes

2 duck breasts, skin on
1 tbsp of Chinese five spice
Olive oil
2 cloves garlic, minced
2 tbsp grated ginger
½ red chilli, sliced
4 cups bone broth (see
  page 245) or vegetable
  stock (see page 243)
5 white mushrooms, sliced
400g canned adzuki
  beans, drained and rinsed
2 tbsp miso paste
2 cups kale, chopped
50g vermicelli noodles

To serve:
Spring onion, sliced
Sesame seeds, toasted
Sliced red chilli or chilli
  flakes
Nori, torn into pieces

Preheat the oven to 190°C fan-forced and line a tray with baking paper.

Place the duck breasts skin side up on the tray and season with Chinese five spice. Bake in the oven for 15-20 minutes or until cooked. Remove and allow to rest for 3 minutes before thinly slicing.

Meanwhile, place a large pot with olive oil over medium heat. Add the garlic, ginger and chilli and sauté for 2 minutes. Add the bone broth or stock, mushrooms and adzuki beans and bring to a simmer for 10 minutes.

In a small bowl, mix the miso paste with a ladle of warm broth until smooth. Stir back into the pot.

Add the kale and noodles to the pot and simmer for another 2-3 minutes, keeping the kale vibrant. Turn off and let the broth sit until the noodles are cooked.

Serve the broth in a bowl and top with the sliced duck. Garnish with spring onions, toasted sesame seeds, fresh chilli/chilli flakes and nori pieces.

**NOTES:**
> If you can only find duck breasts premarinated in peking duck sauce, omit the Chinese five spice.
> For ease of eating, precook the noodles in a separate pot and cut into pieces using scissors, then add to the broth.

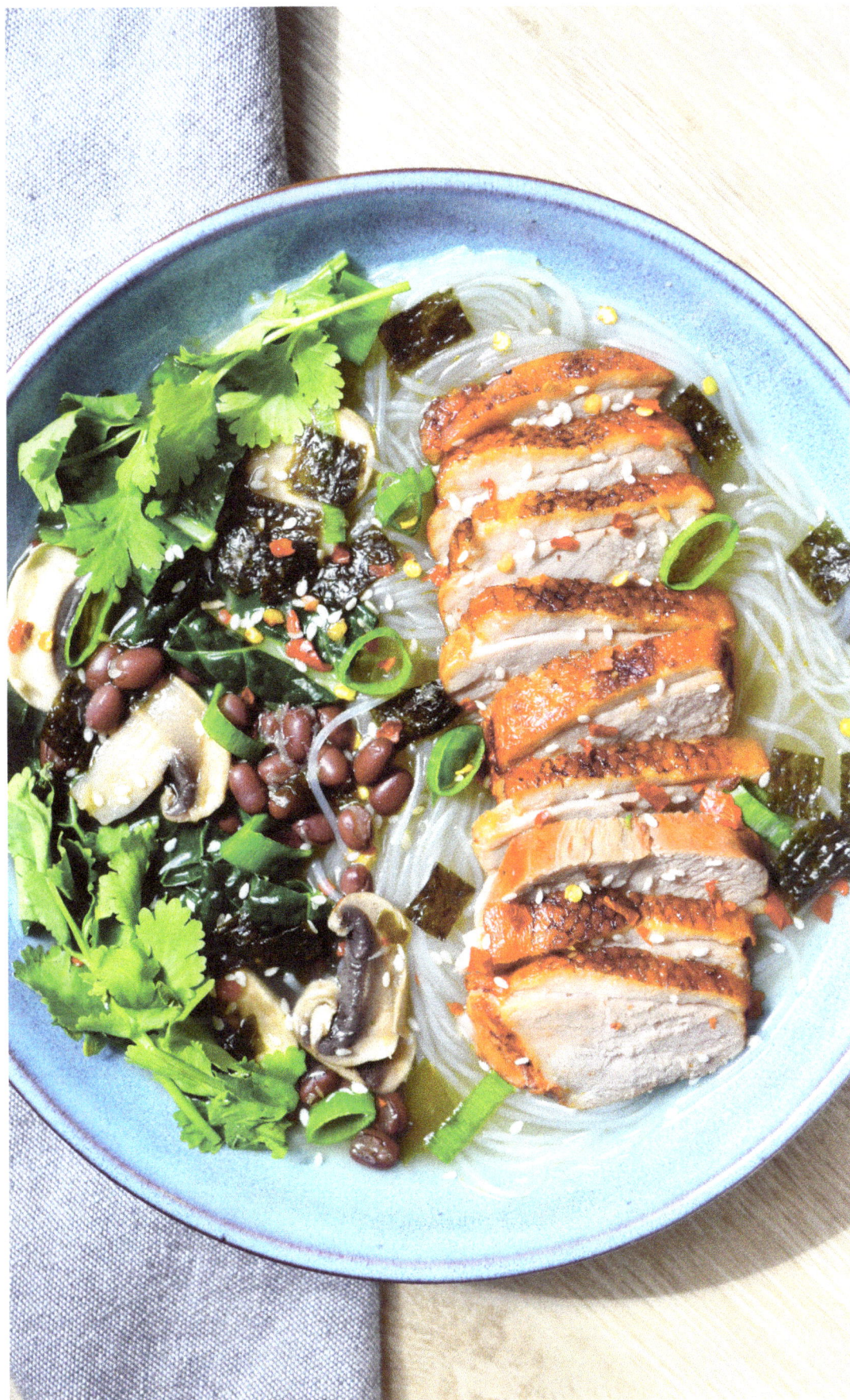

# PRAWN RED CURRY

**Serves:** 2     **Prep:** 10 minutes     **Cook:** 15 minutes

Olive oil
2 tbsp fresh ginger, grated
2 cloves garlic, grated
1 green chilli, sliced
2 tbsp red curry paste
2 tbsp miso paste
1 cup water
1 red capsicum, diced
1 tomato, chopped
400ml coconut milk
2 tbsp fish sauce
1 tbsp maple syrup
1 lime, juiced
200g prawns, shelled and
   deveined
2 cups kale, chopped

**To serve:**
2 cups wild rice, cooked

**To garnish (optional):**
Sliced green chilli
Coriander
Spring onion, sliced
Lime wedges

Heat a pan or wok to medium and drizzle some olive oil. Add the ginger, garlic and green chilli and cook for a further 2 minutes.

Then add the red curry paste, miso paste and a cup of water, cooking for 2 minutes until fragrant.

Add the capsicum, tomato, coconut milk, fish sauce, maple syrup and lime juice to the pan and cook for 5 minutes. Add the prawns and cook for 10 minutes.

Once the prawns are cooked, add the kale and stir through, allowing it to wilt.

Serve with wild rice and garnish with sliced green chilli, coriander, spring onion and a lime wedge (if desired).

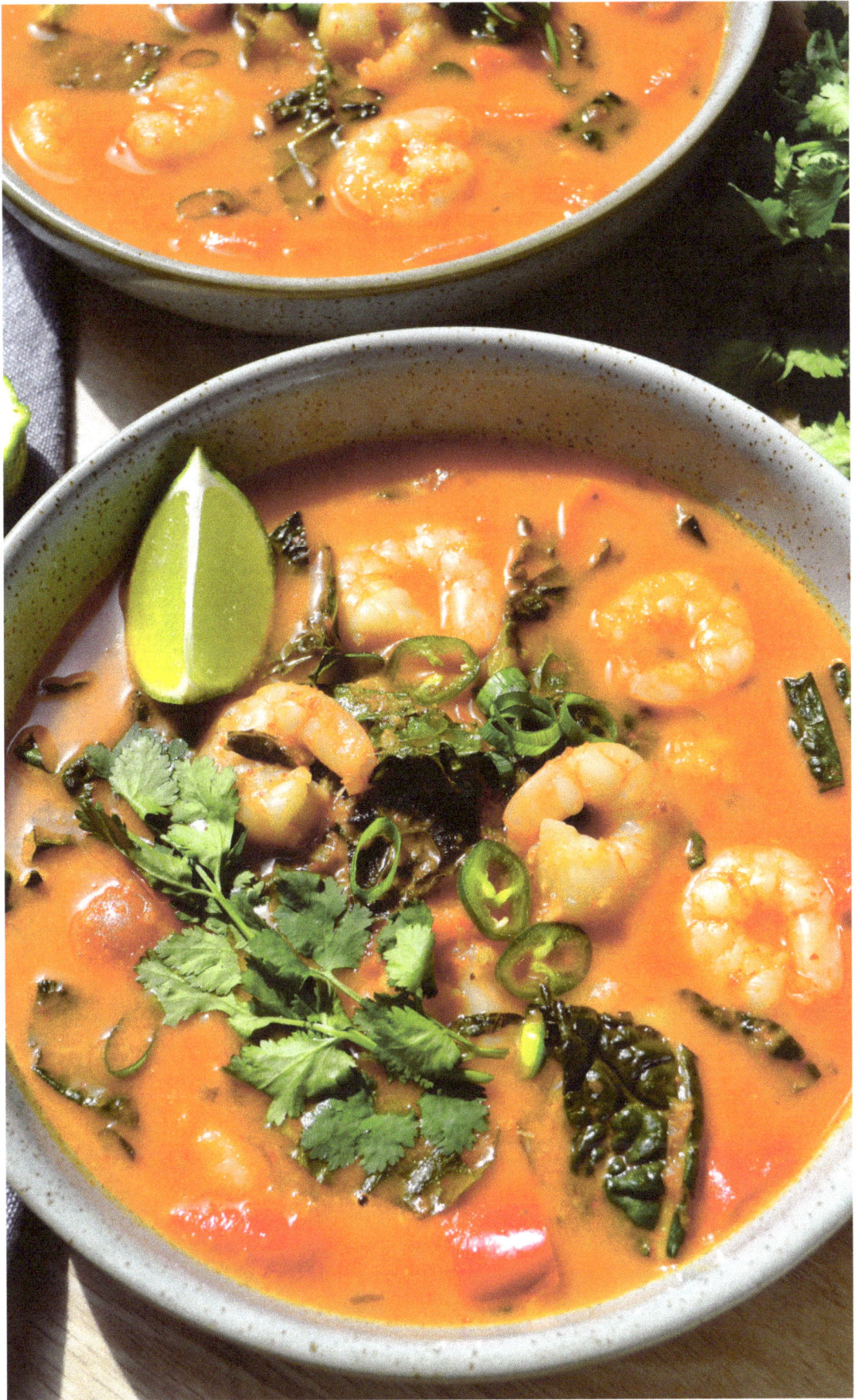

# snacks

Hazelnut Bliss Balls

Beetroot Dip

Beetroot &
Black Bean Brownies

Buckwheat Bars

Choc-Orange Mousse
with Blueberry Compote

Sardine Bruschetta

# HAZELNUT BLISS BALLS

**Serves:** 10-12 pieces  **Prep:** 10 minutes  **Cook:** 1 hour

6 medjool dates, pitted
2 tbsp peanut butter
1 tbsp chia seeds
2 tbsp hazelnuts
1 tbsp cacao powder
1 tbsp water
½ cup crushed peanuts

Place the dates, peanut butter, chia seeds, half of the hazelnuts, cacao powder and water into a food processor. Blend until combined.

With damp hands, take a heaped teaspoon of the mixture and roll into balls. Place 1 hazelnut into the centre and continue rolling until the hazelnut is covered. Repeat the process with the remaining mixture.

Coat the balls in the crushed peanuts.

Refrigerate to set for at least 1 hour.

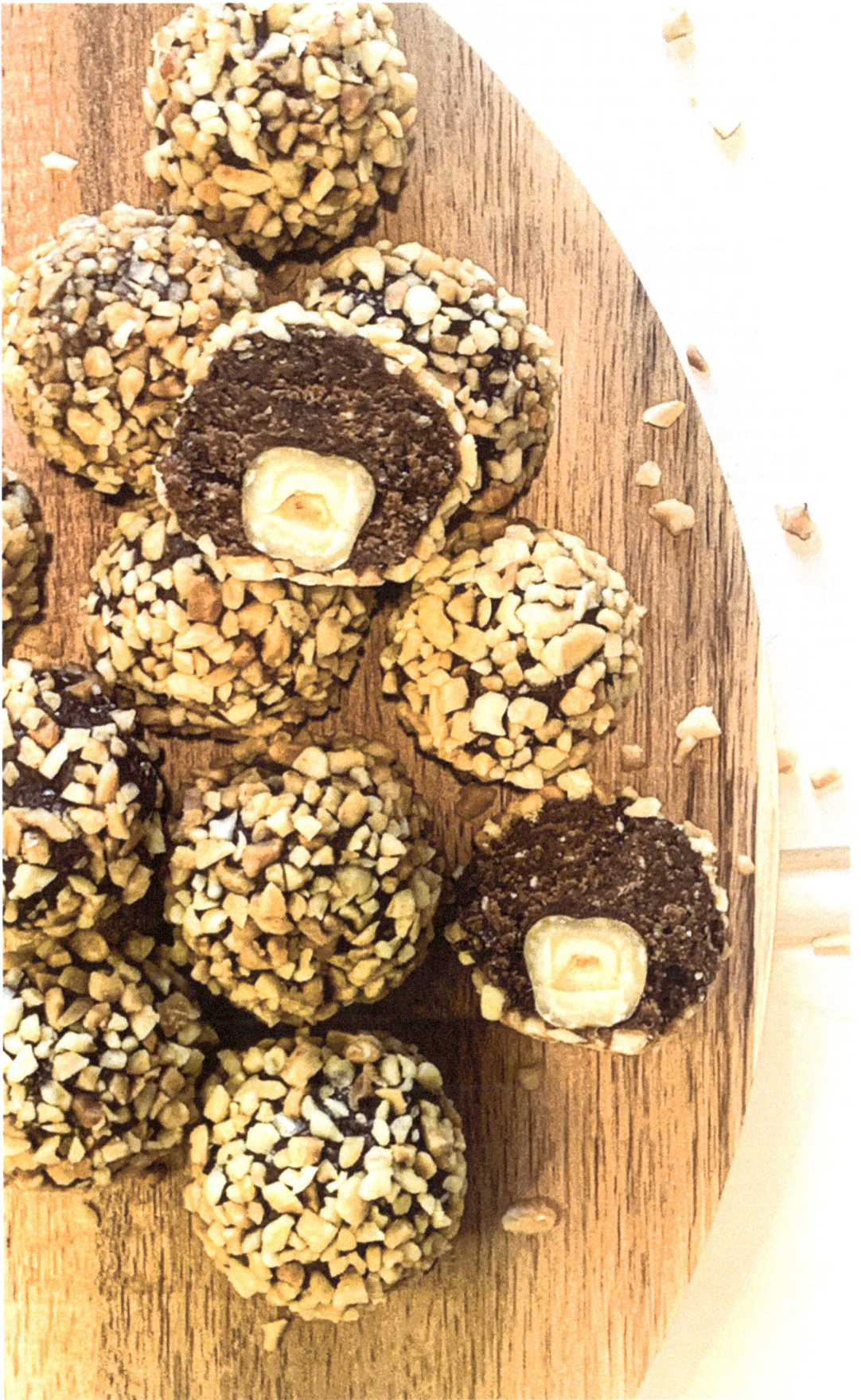

# BEETROOT DIP

**Serves:** 2     **Prep:** 5 minutes     **Cook:** 1 minute

425g canned baby
  beetroots, drained and
  rinsed
400g canned red kidney
  beans, drained and rinsed
½ cup fresh mint
½ cup natural Greek
  yoghurt
¼ cup sunflower seeds
1 tsp cumin
1 lemon, juiced

Add all the ingredients to a food processor and blend until the mixture is smooth.

Serve with veggie sticks and/or seed crackers of your choice.

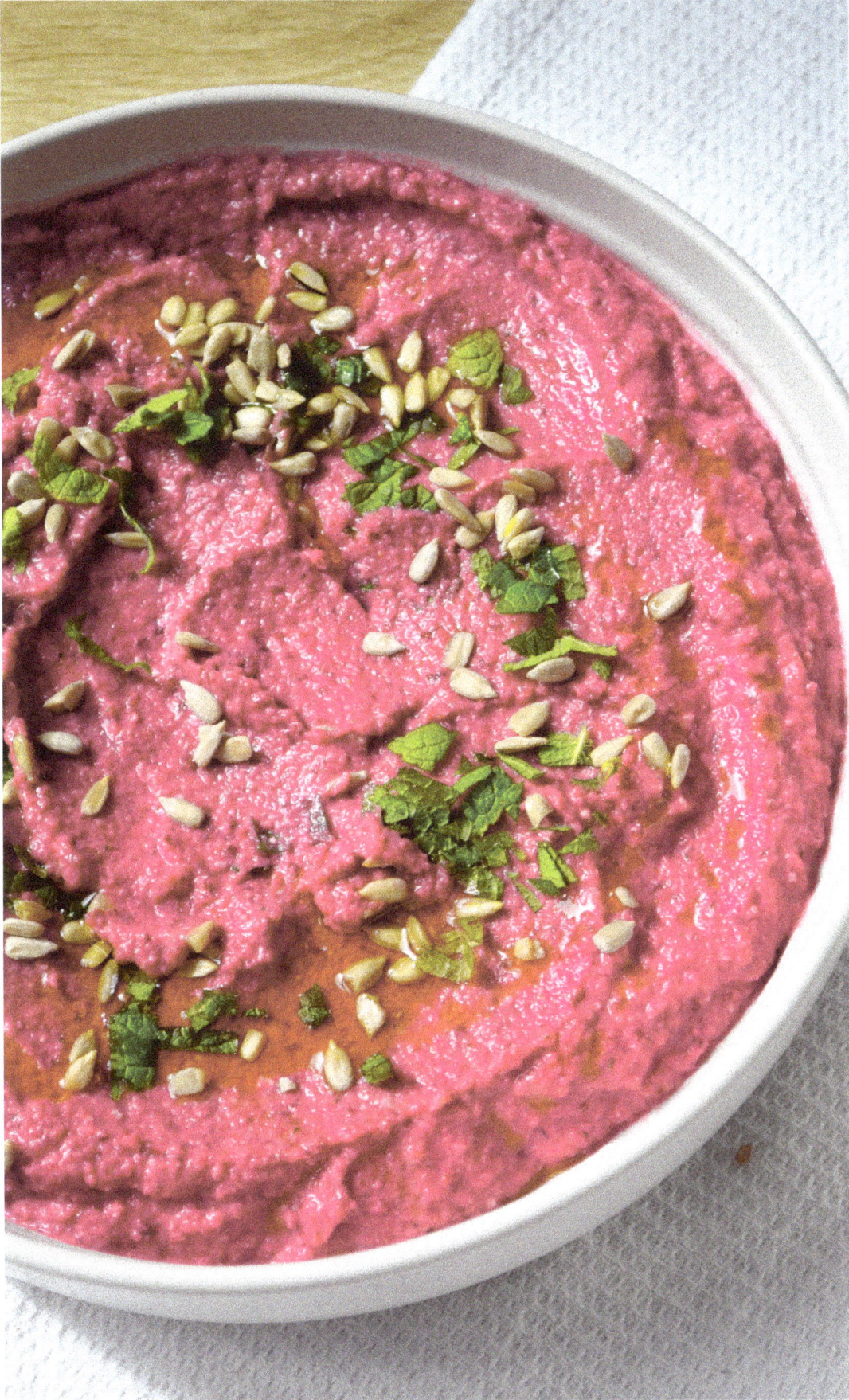

# BEETROOT & BLACK BEAN BROWNIES

**Serves:** 16      **Prep:** 5 minutes      **Cook:** 40 minutes

1 beetroot, peeled and
  diced
400g black beans, drained
  and rinsed
3 tbsp flaxseed meal
3 tbsp cacao powder
1 tbsp maple syrup
½ tsp baking soda
3 tbsp tahini
3 tbsp coconut oil
⅓ cup almond flour*
2 tbsp chia seeds
1 tbsp protein powder
  of choice (vanilla or
  unsweetened)
2 tbsp water
¼ cup dark chocolate,
  roughly chopped
¼ cup walnuts, roughly
  chopped

Pre-heat the oven to 180°C fan-forced and line a 20x20cm
baking dish.

Steam the diced beetroot for 10 minutes or until tender using
a steaming basket over a pot of boiling water.

In a food processor, combine all the ingredients, except
the dark chocolate pieces and walnuts, and blend
until smooth.

Add the mixture to the lined baking dish and spread it
out evenly.

Top with the dark chocolate pieces and walnuts and bake
in the oven for 25 minutes.

Remove from the oven and allow to sit for 15 minutes before
slicing into squares.

Store in the refrigerator until ready to eat.

*Recipe gives between 5-6g protein per square.*

**NOTE:**
› Blend ¼ cup of almonds to make almond flour.

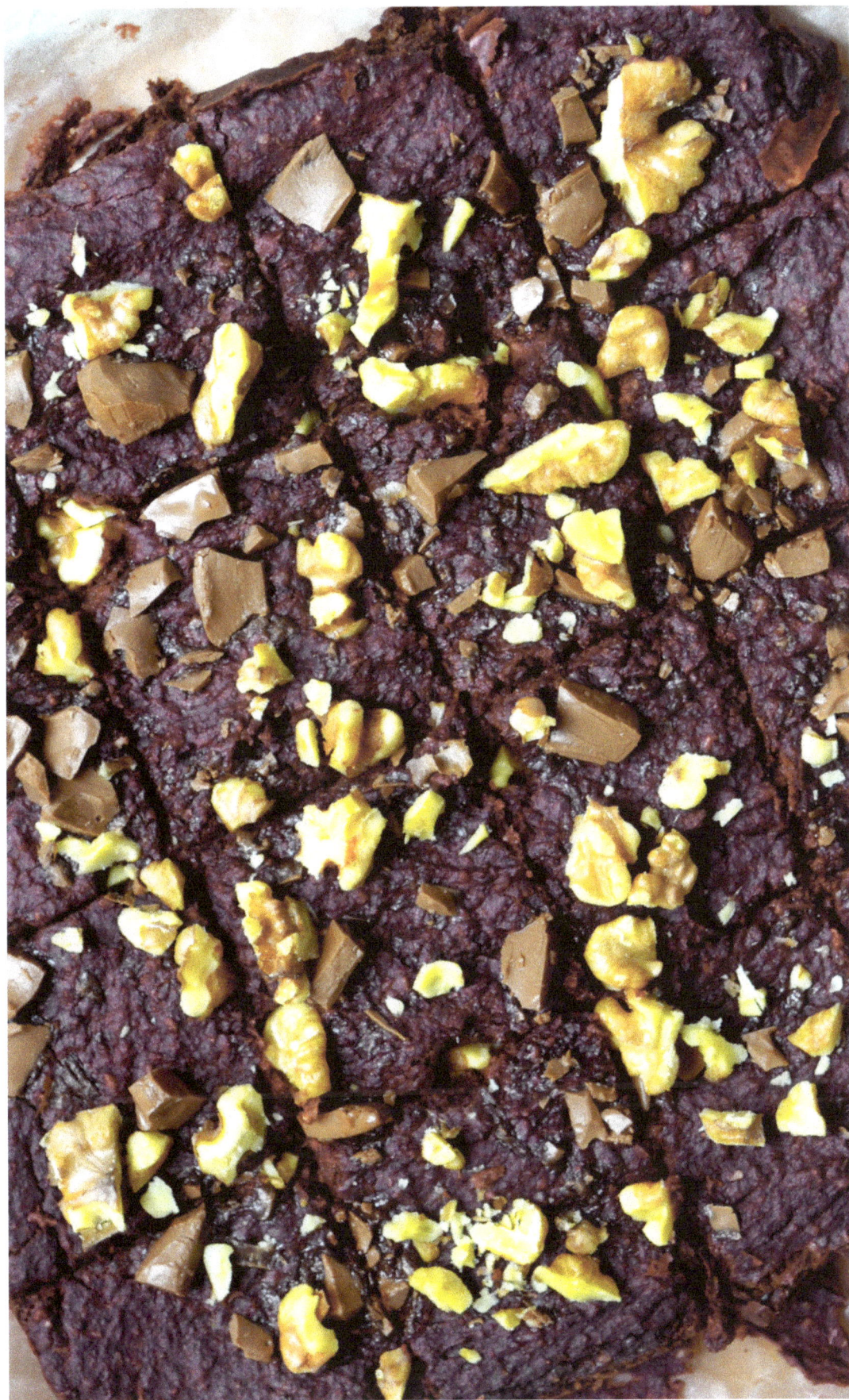

# BUCKWHEAT BARS

**Serves:** 8     **Prep:** 5 minutes     **Cook:** 45 minutes

6 medjool dates, pitted
1 cup buckwheat groats
½ cup oats
1 tbsp flaxseed meal
1 tbsp maple syrup
¼ cup coconut oil, melted
1 tsp vanilla extract
¼ cup dark chocolate
  pieces (add more if
  desired)

Preheat the oven to 180°C fan-forced and line a
bread loaf tin.

In a food processor, add the dates and blend. Add the
buckwheat, oats and flaxseed meal, then blend again.

Add the maple syrup, melted coconut oil and vanilla extract
to the buckwheat mixture. Blend until all the ingredients are
combined. Stir in the dark chocolate pieces.

Transfer the mixture to the bread tin, pressing it out evenly.
With a knife, slice the pressed mixture into bars.

Bake in the oven for 30 minutes. Remove from the oven,
gently separate the pieces and place them on a larger tray.
Continue baking for an additional 10-15 minutes until the
bars are crispy.

Remove from the oven and allow to cool.

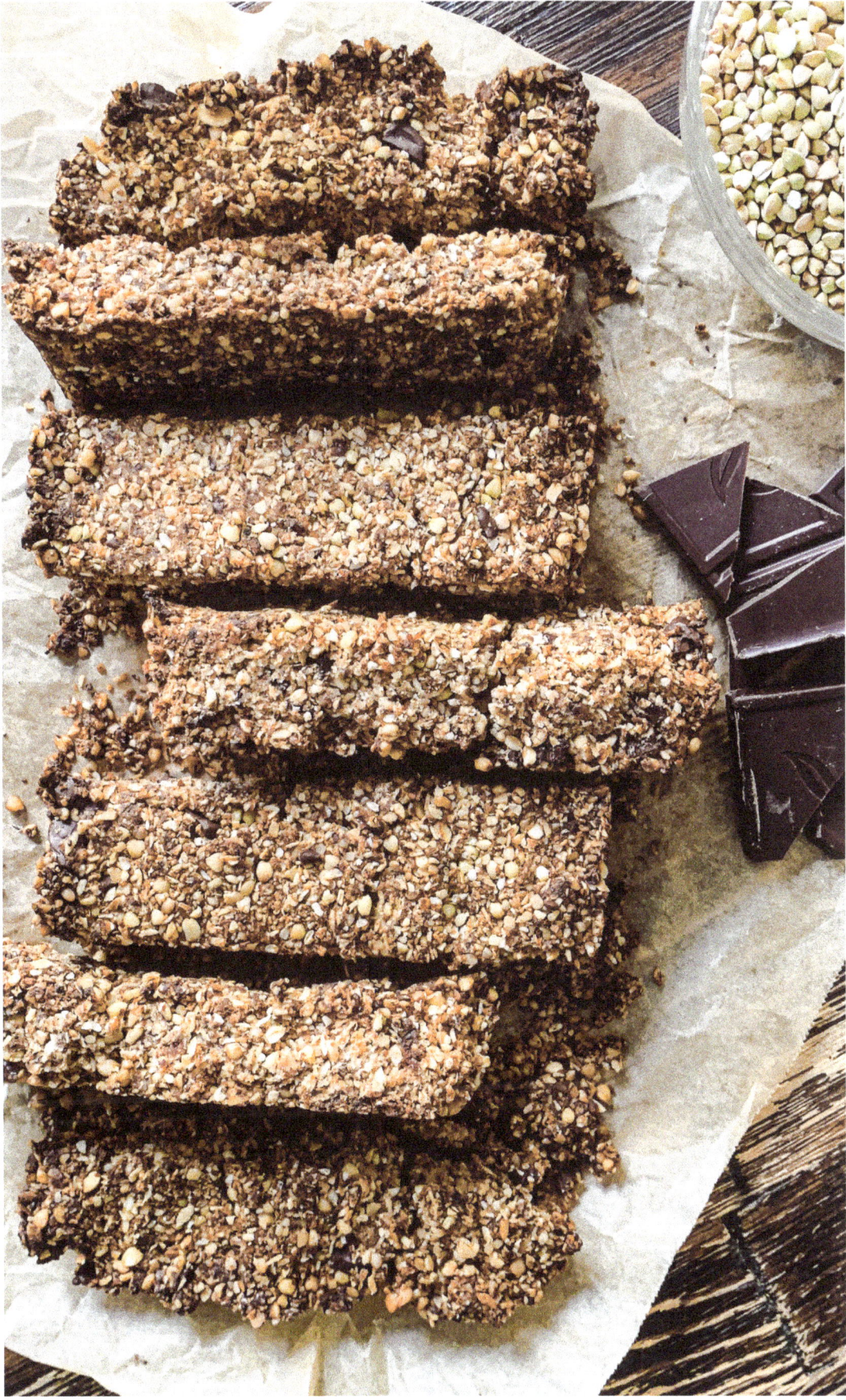

# CHOC-ORANGE MOUSSE
## WITH BLUEBERRY COMPOTE

**Serves:** 2     **Prep:** 5 minutes     **Cook:** 30 minutes

1 cup cottage cheese
½ cup vanilla flavoured
   Greek yoghurt
1 egg
1 tbsp cacao powder
1 tsp maple syrup
½ tsp vanilla extract
1 orange, juiced and zested
½ cup frozen blueberries
3 tbsp water

Preheat the oven to 180°C fan-forced.

In a food processor, add the cottage cheese, yoghurt, egg, cacao, maple syrup, vanilla extract and half of the orange juice. Blend until a smooth and creamy texture has formed.

Add to 2 ramekin dishes and bake in the oven for 25–30 minutes, or until the mixture has solidified and cracks begin to form.

Meanwhile, add the blueberries, the other half of the orange juice and water to a small pot and simmer on a low heat for about 5 minutes, until the berries have softened and the water is a deep purple.

Once the mousse has cooked, serve by topping with the blueberry compote and a sprinkle of the orange zest.

This is best served warm (to be supportive of the menstrual phase, but can also be enjoyed cold).

This recipe can also be enjoyed in the late luteal phase.

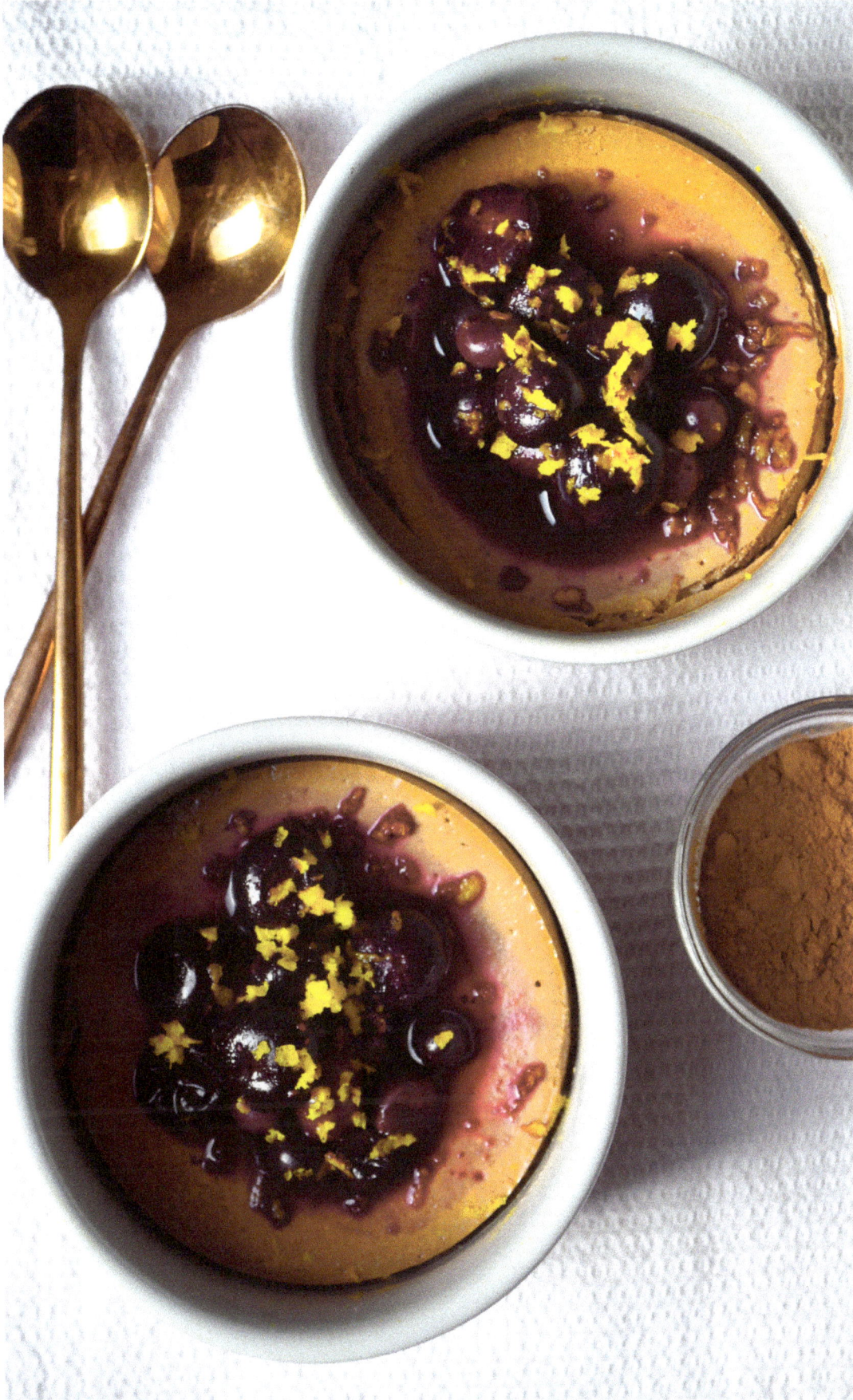

# SARDINE BRUSCHETTA

**Serves:** 1     **Prep:** 5 minutes     **Cook:** N/A

1 tomato, diced
1 tbsp basil or parsley, chopped
1 garlic clove (optional)
½ red onion, finely chopped
1 tsp olive oil
1 tbsp tomato paste
2 pieces of sourdough bread, toasted or fresh
1 tin sardines (or smoked oysters)

In a small bowl, combine the diced tomatoes, basil, garlic, red onion and oil.

Spread the tomato paste on the toast. Add the sardine fillets and top with the tomato and onion mix.

Drizzle with additional olive oil if desired.

Serve immediately.

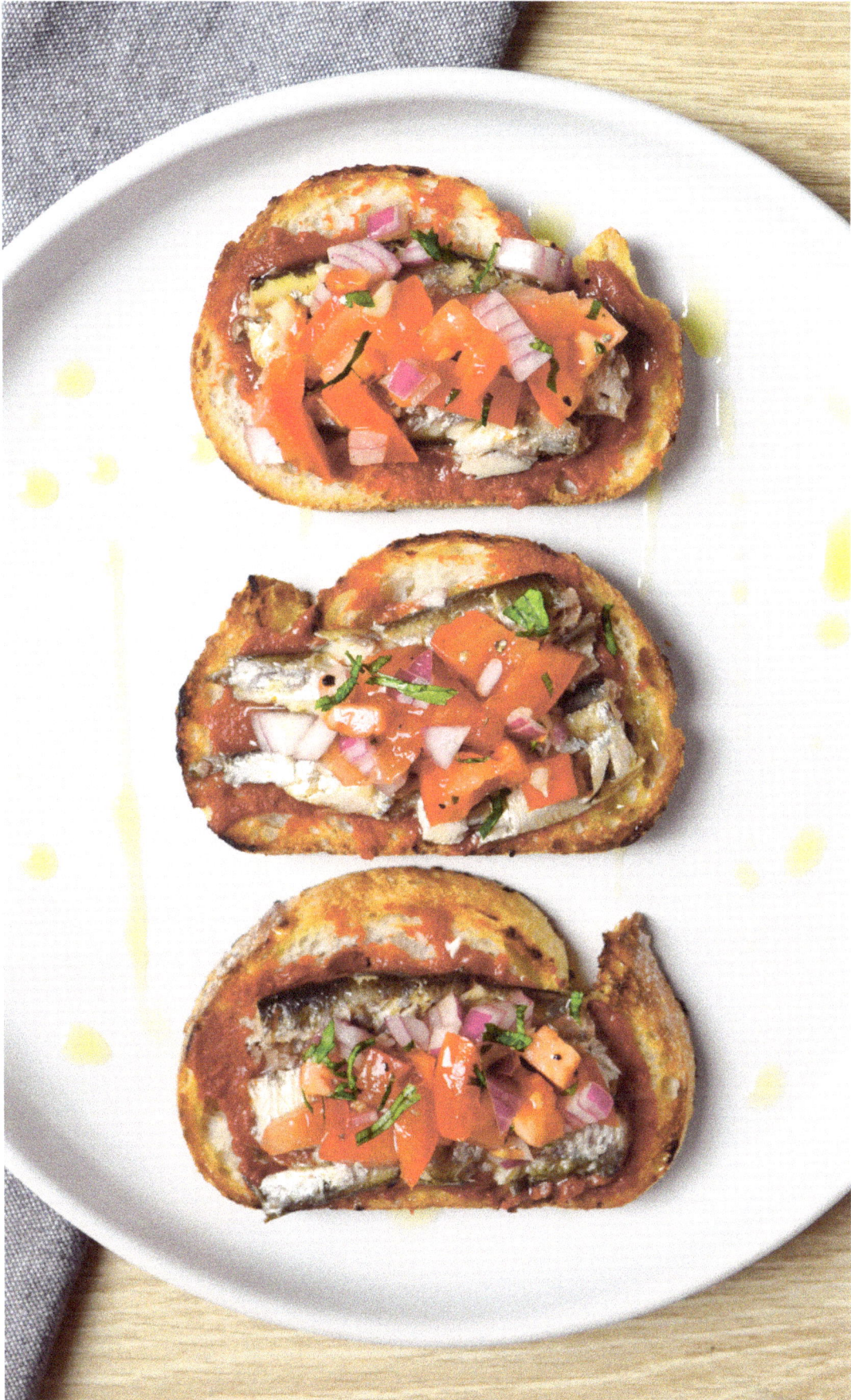

# follicular phase

# HERO FOODS

**NUTRIENTS FOR THE FOLLICULAR PHASE**

ZINC | CALCIUM | SELENIUM | B-VITAMINS

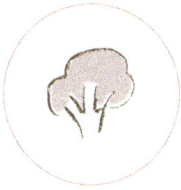

BROCCOLI

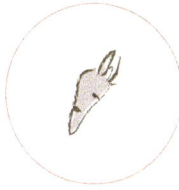

CARROT

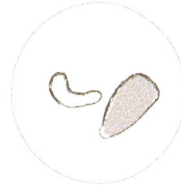

NUTS
(CASHEWS & BRAZIL)

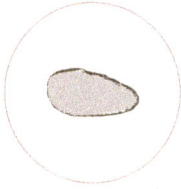

CHICKEN

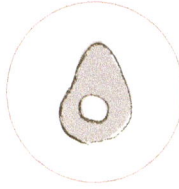

AVOCADO

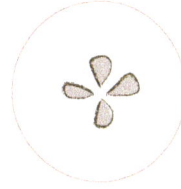

CITRUS FRUITS

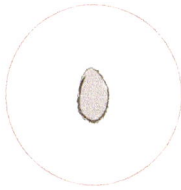

EGGS

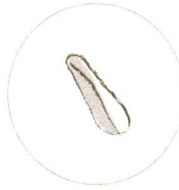

ZUCCHINI

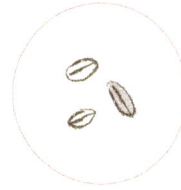

OATS

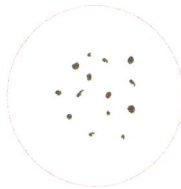

SEEDS
(PUMPKIN & FLAX)

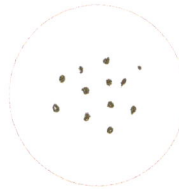

LENTILS

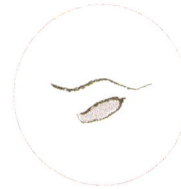

FERMENTED FOODS

*follicular recipes*

# breakfast

Growth &
Energy Smoothie

Baked Oats

Green Goddess
Shakshuka

Lemon Cheesecake
Overnight Weetbix

Loaded Protein
Smashed Avo

Turkish Eggs

Choc Cherry
Overnight Oats

# GROWTH & ENERGY SMOOTHIE

**Serves:** 1     **Prep:** 5 minutes     **Cook:** N/A

1 cup baby spinach
½ avocado
1 green apple
1 tbsp flaxseeds
½ cup cucumber, diced
1 cup coconut water
1 tsp spirulina or
  chlorella (optional)
1 tbsp pumpkin seeds
1 heaped tbsp protein
  powder
1 tbsp mint
½ lime, juiced

Add all the ingredients into a blender and blend until smooth. Serve immediately.

*This recipe also doubles as a snack option.*

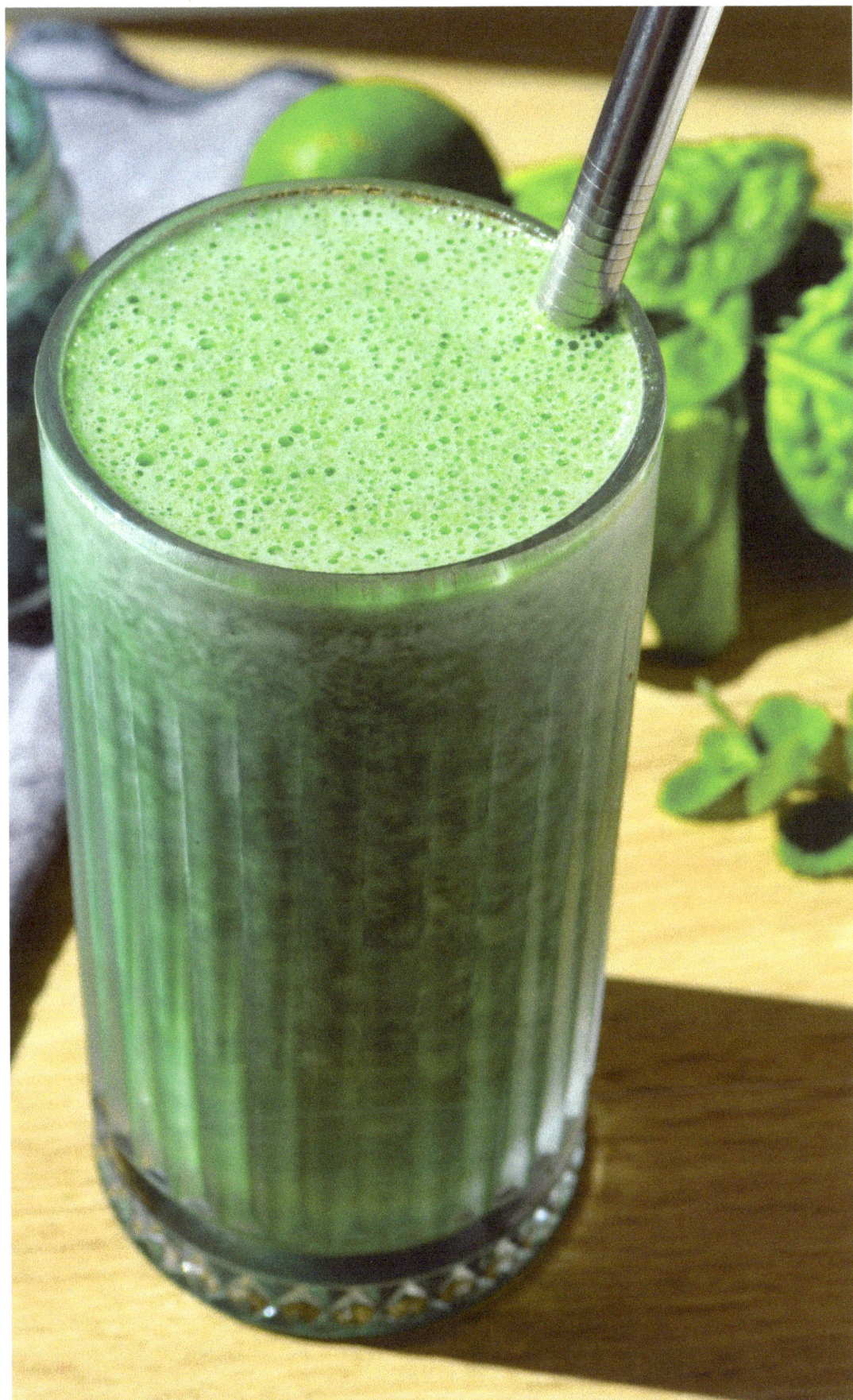

# BAKED OATS

**Serves:** 4    **Prep:** 5 minutes    **Cook:** 40 minutes

2 bananas, mashed
2 cups oats
4 heaped tbsp vanilla
  protein powder
¼ cup chia seeds
400ml coconut milk
1 cup frozen cherries

**To serve:**
140g Greek yoghurt (per
  serve)
Nut butter of choice
  (optional)

Preheat the oven to 180°C fan-forced.

In a 20x20cm baking dish, add the mashed bananas. Then add the oats, protein powder, chia seeds and coconut milk. Mix together to combine. Evenly distribute mixture over the base of the tray. Top with frozen cherries.

Bake in the oven for 30-40 minutes or until the oats are golden brown.

Serve with Greek yoghurt and a drizzle of nut butter.

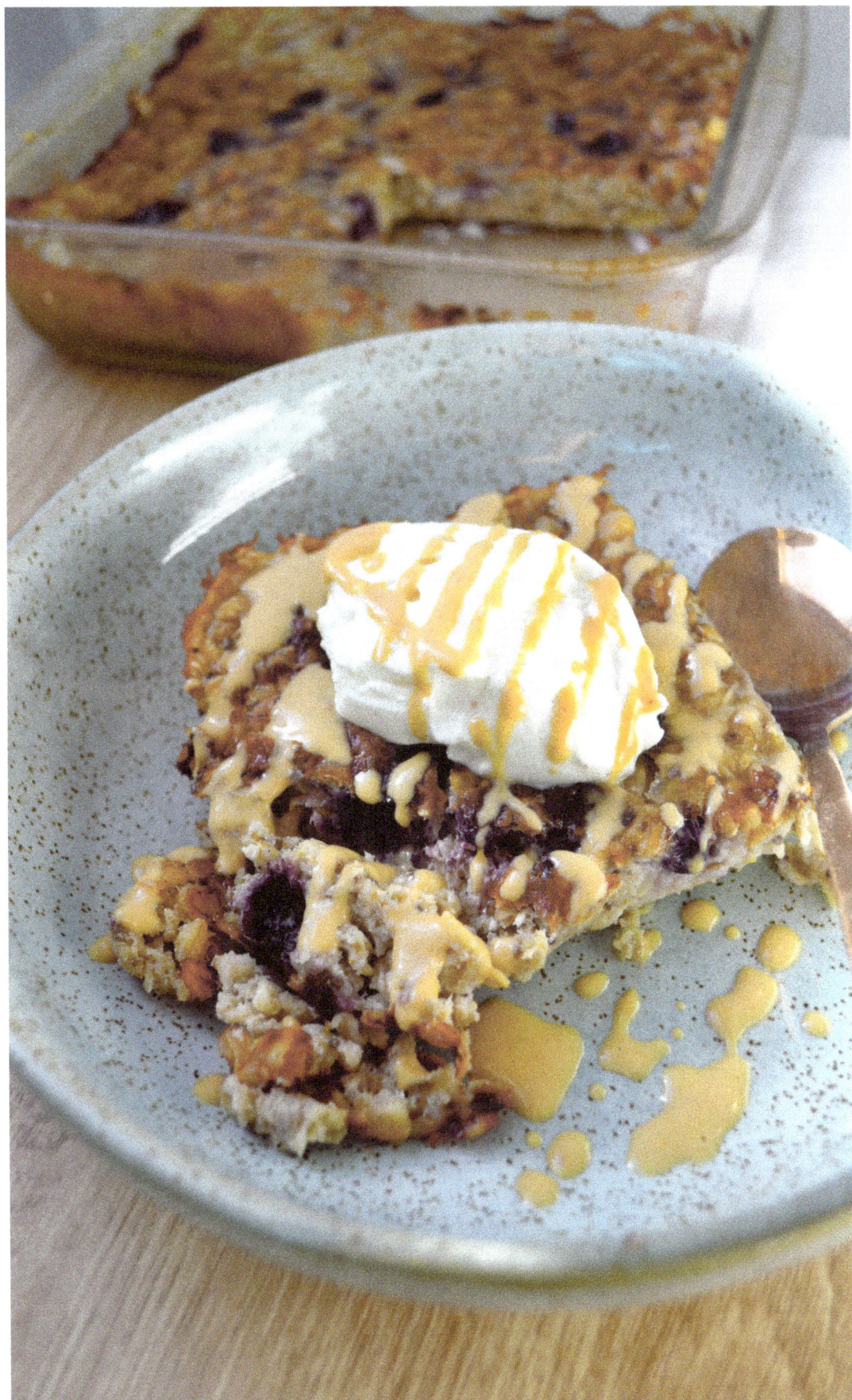

# GREEN GODDESS SHAKSHUKA

**Serves:** 4     **Prep:** 10 minutes     **Cook:** 15 minutes

**For the green goddess sauce:**
1 avocado
½ cup parsley, tightly packed
½ cup dill, tightly packed
1 cup spinach
1 zucchini, chopped
1 ½ cups cottage cheese
¼ cup milk
¼ cup hemp seeds
¼ cup water
1 tbsp Dijon mustard

**For the shakshuka:**
½ tsp olive oil
1 white onion/shallot, finely diced
2 garlic cloves, finely chopped
1 bunch broccolini, chopped into fifths
1 bunch asparagus, chopped into fifths
½ cup frozen green peas
6 eggs
¼ cup feta cheese, crumbled (optional)

**To serve:**
Sourdough toast

In a blender, add all the ingredients for the green goddess sauce. Blend until a smooth, creamy texture has formed. Set aside.

Heat a large pan on medium and add the olive oil. Add the onion and garlic and sauté for 2-3 minutes until softened. Add the broccolini, asparagus and peas. Sauté for another 2 minutes to allow the greens to become tender.

Add the green goddess sauce to the pan and stir well to combine the greens with the sauce. Allow to simmer for 5 minutes, stirring continuously.

Create 6 wells in the sauce and crack the eggs into them. Top with feta cheese and cover on a medium-low heat until the eggs are cooked to your preference.

Garnish with extra herbs and feta and serve with toasted sourdough, if desired.

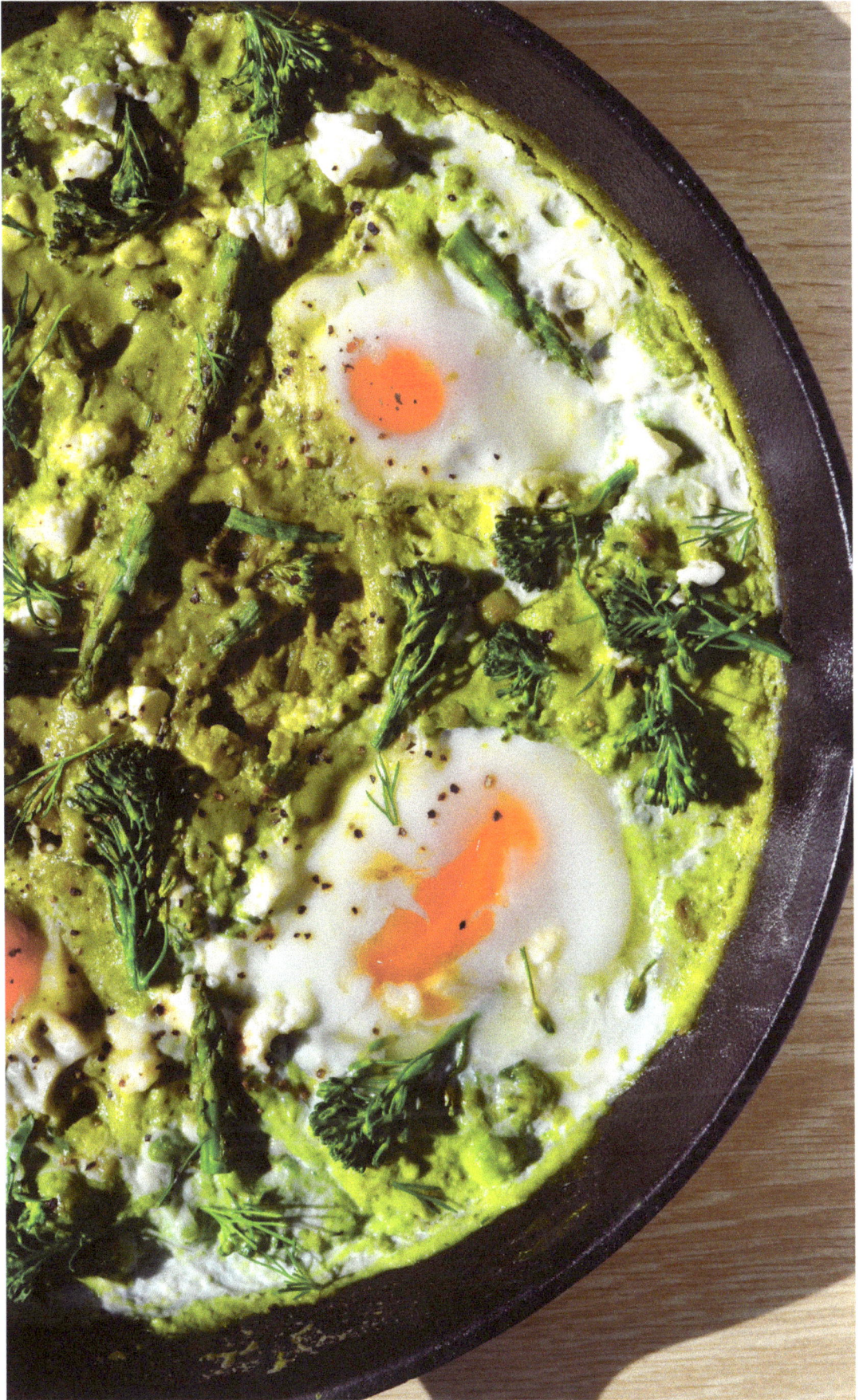

# LEMON CHEESECAKE OVERNIGHT WEETBIX

**Serves:** 2     **Prep:** 5 minutes     **Cook:** 2 hours +

**For the base:**
4 Weetbix
1 cup water
2 tbsp chia seeds
1 tbsp lemon zest
1 lemon, juiced

**For the centre:**
1 banana, sliced

**For the topping:**
1 cup vanilla protein yoghurt
  OR Greek yoghurt + 1 tbsp
  vanilla protein
2 tbsp cashews
2 tbsp pepita seeds

**To garnish (optional):**
Lemon slices
Lemon zest

In 2 glass containers, add 2 Weetbix biscuits and crush them into small pieces. Divide and combine the remaining base ingredients between the two containers. Smooth the surface and then add the sliced banana. Refrigerate while making the other layers.

In a blender, add the cashews and pepita seeds and blend to create a "crumble-like" texture. Set aside.

Remove containers from the fridge. Top base with yoghurt and smooth the surface to create an even layer. Sprinkle the nut and seed crumb on, then top with lemon slices and zest if desired.

Place in the fridge to set for at least 2 hours.

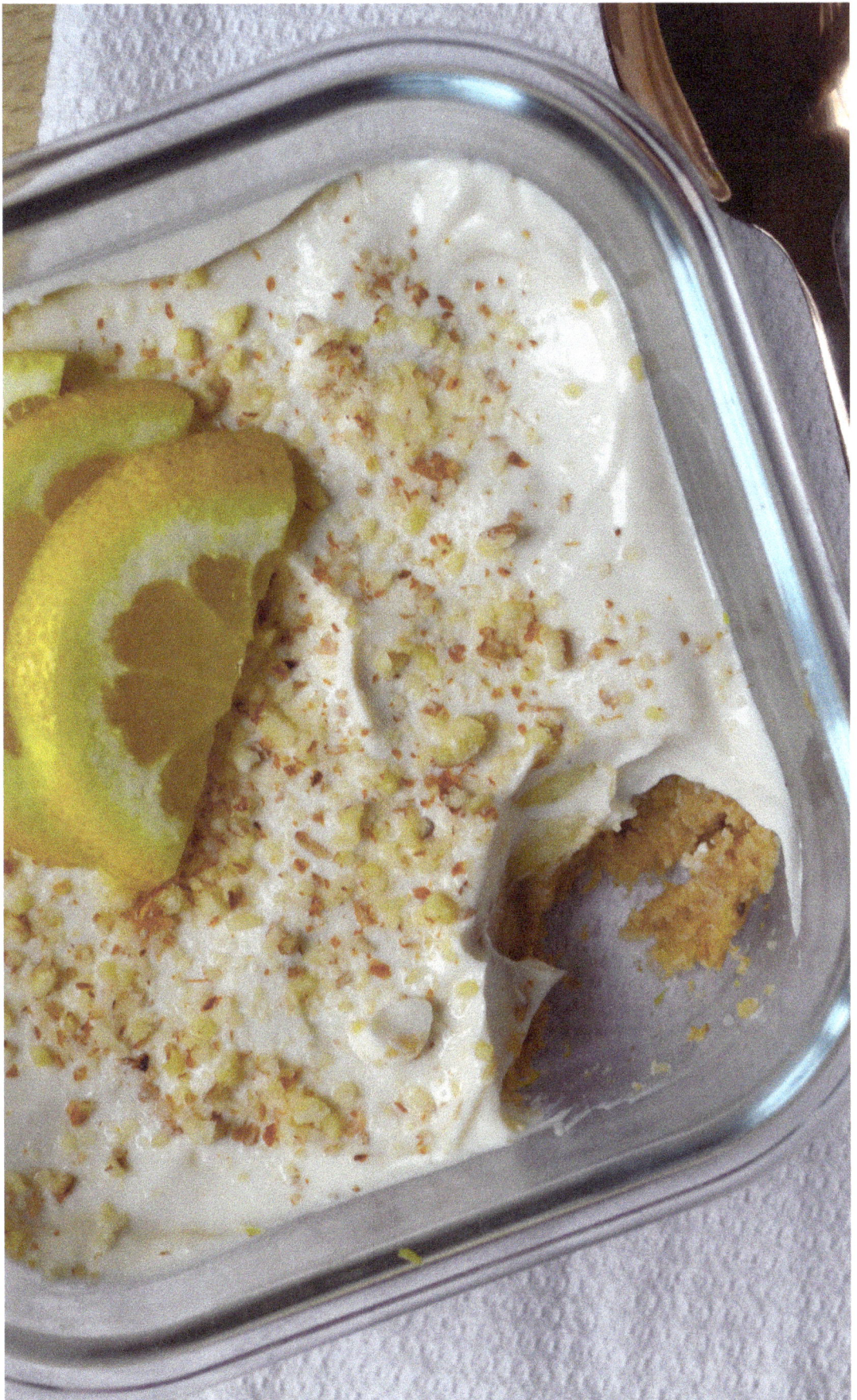

# LOADED PROTEIN SMASHED AVO

**Serves:** 2     **Prep:** 5 minutes     **Cook:** N/A

1 avocado
200g canned cannellini
  beans, drained and rinsed
½ lemon, juiced
1 tsp olive oil
½ tsp ground cumin
  (optional)
Salt and pepper, to season
Chilli flakes, to garnish
  (optional)

**Add extra protein:**
½ cup cottage cheese
2 hard boiled eggs, finely
  chopped

**To serve:**
Sourdough bread

In a bowl, mash the avocado and beans together using a fork or potato masher. Add in the cottage cheese or chopped boiled eggs for additional protein, if desired.

Mix in the lemon juice, olive oil and cumin, if using, and season with salt and pepper.

Serve on toasted bread and garnish with chilli flakes.

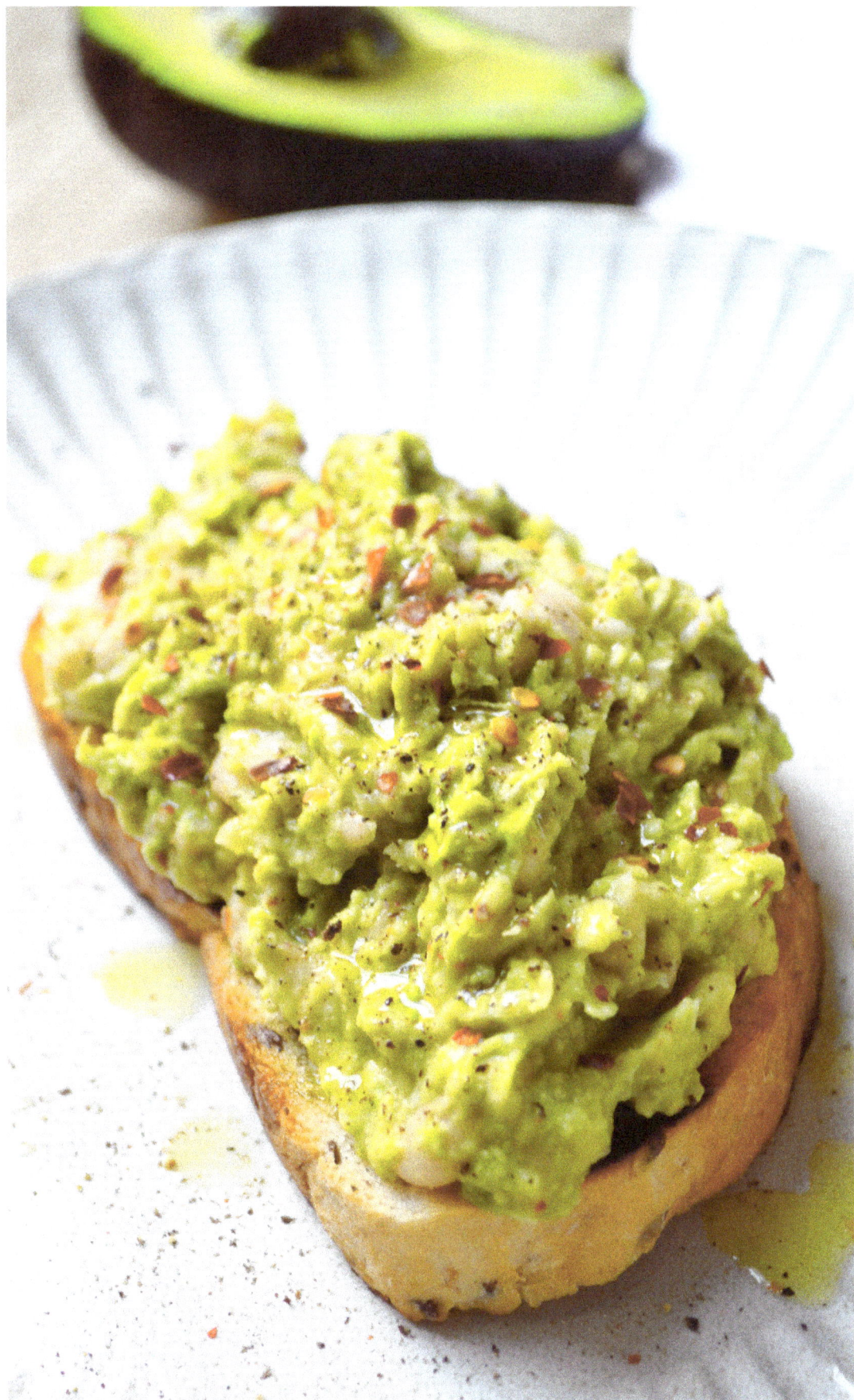

# TURKISH EGGS

**Serves:** 4    **Prep:** 5 minutes    **Cook:** 10 minutes

8 eggs
4 cups Greek yoghurt
2 garlic cloves, grated
⅓ cup dill, chopped
¼ cup olive oil
1 tbsp paprika
⅛ tsp cayenne pepper

To serve:
Sourdough bread

Bring a pot of water to boil. Add the eggs and boil for 7 minutes (for a soft boiled egg). Remove eggs from pot and add to a bowl of cold water. Peel eggs and set aside until ready to serve.

Meanwhile, combine the yoghurt, garlic and dill in a bowl. Set aside.

In a heated pan, add the olive oil, paprika and cayenne pepper, cook for about a minute.

Assemble the dish by placing the yoghurt in bowls and topping with the boiled eggs. Drizzle the chilli oil and garnish with more dill (if desired).

Serve with sourdough bread.

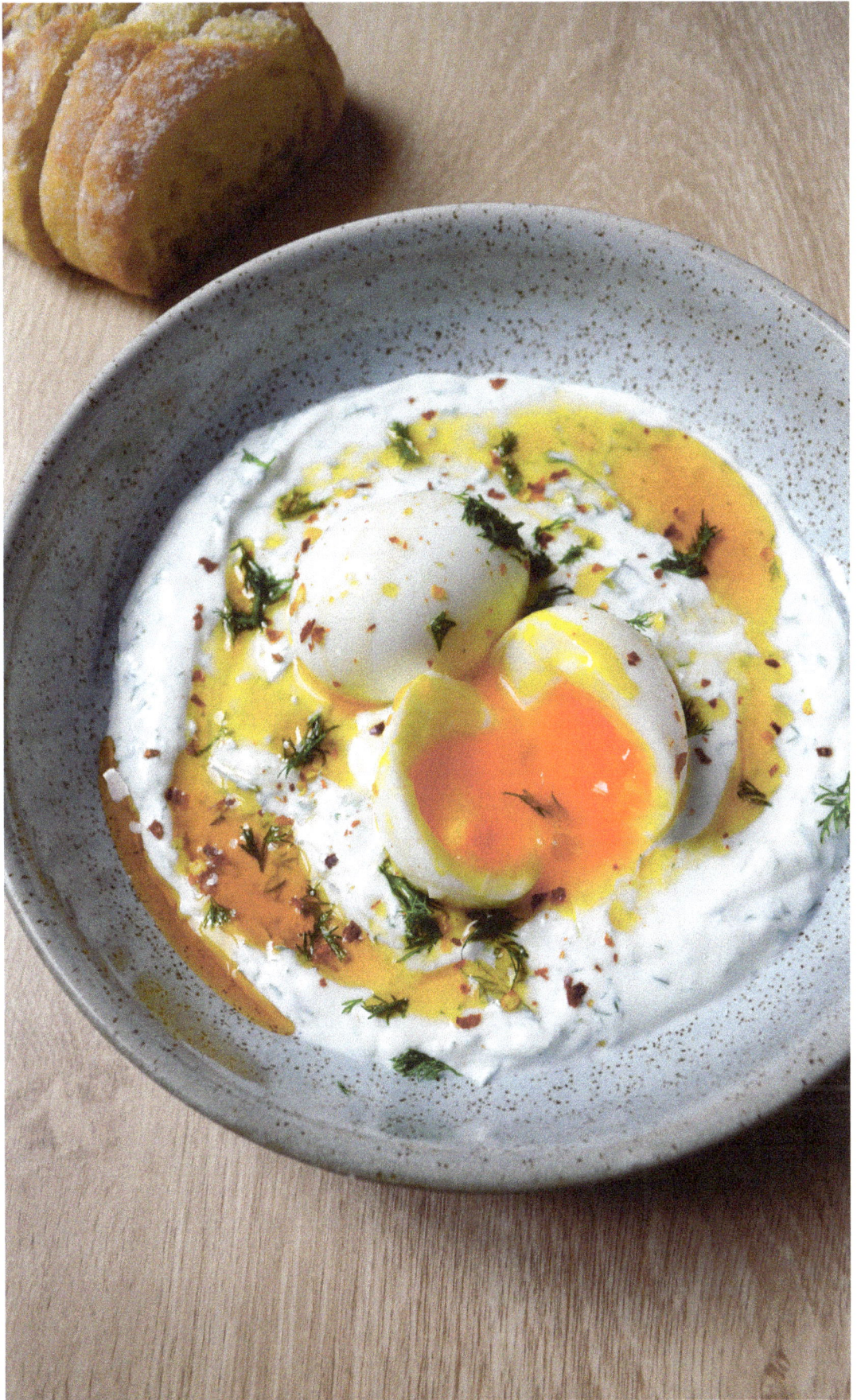

# CHOC CHERRY OVERNIGHT OATS

**Serves:** 2    **Prep:** 5 minutes    **Cook:** 2 hours +

1 cup rolled oats
1 cup kefir
2 tbsp chia seeds
½ cup frozen cherries

**For the topping:**
1 tbsp cacao
1 tbsp coconut oil, melted
1 tbsp shredded coconut

Add the oats, kefir, chia seeds and cherries into a blender and blend until smooth. Pour into 2 jars or glass containers. Set aside.

In a bowl, combine the cacao and coconut oil until smooth. Pour over the top of the oat mixture.

Top with the shredded coconut.

Refrigerate for at least 2 hours or overnight.

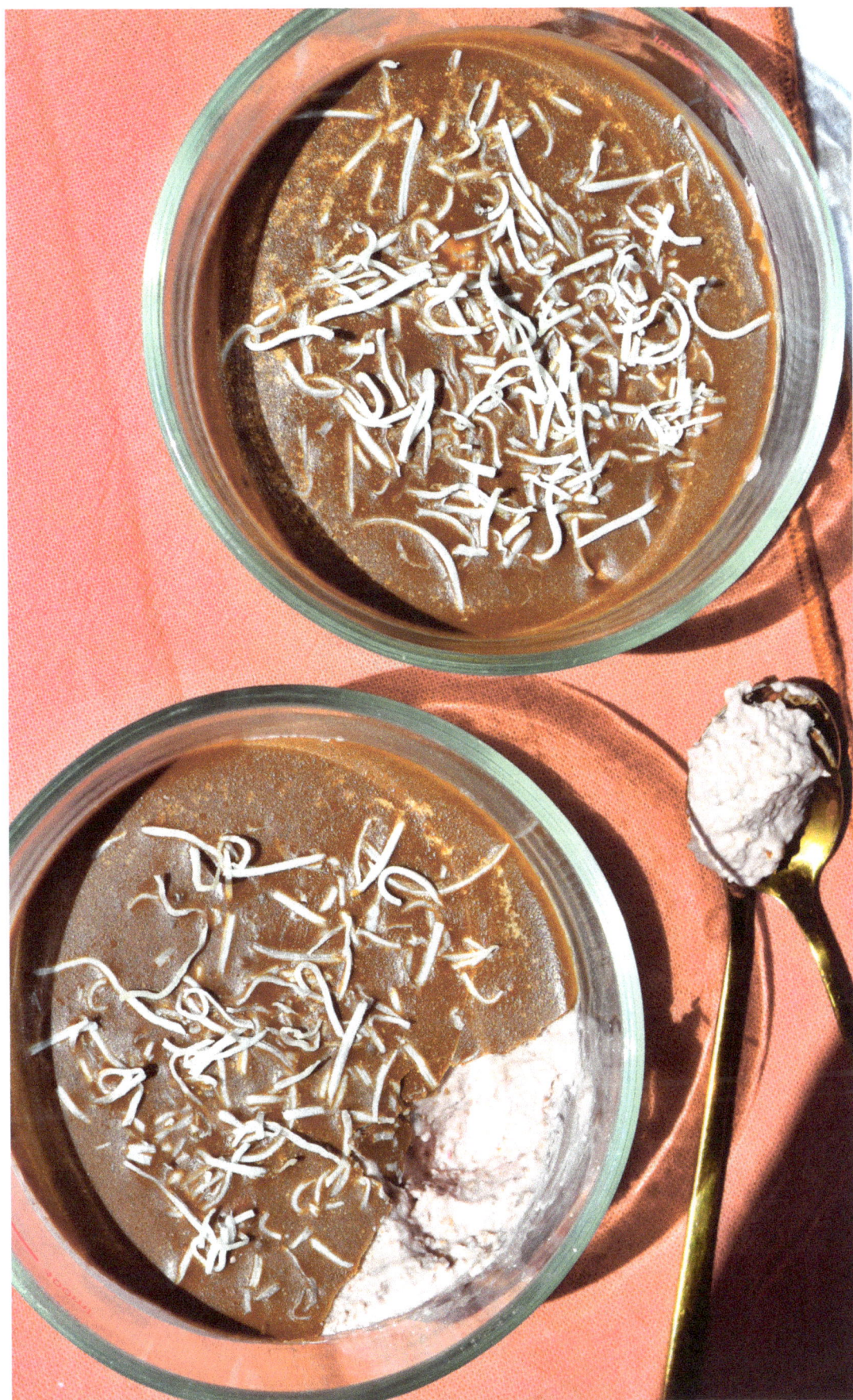

# mains

Lemon Pepper Chicken &
Greens Nourish Bowl

Chicken Noodle &
Vegetable Soup

Follicular Phase
Buddha Bowl

Chicken Pesto Pasta

Springtime Stirfry

Poached Chicken
with Raw Veggie Salad &
Satay Dressing

Nourish Plates

Greek Nourish
Bowls

Lentil &
Parsley Salad

Lemon Pepper Chicken
with Mashed Peas &
Tomato Sauce

# LEMON PEPPER CHICKEN & GREENS NOURISH BOWL

**Serves:** 2  **Prep:** 30 minutes  **Cook:** 30 minutes

3 tbsp olive oil
1 tbsp parsley, chopped
1 tsp pepper
1 tsp Dijon mustard
2 lemons, juiced
2 chicken breasts
1 zucchini, sliced
1 head broccoli/broccolini
2 garlic cloves, crushed
1 cup snow peas, julienned
1 avocado, sliced
1 cup quinoa, cooked
2 tbsp pumpkin seeds

Preheat the oven to 180°C fan-forced.

To make the marinade, add 1 tbsp olive oil, parsley, pepper, Dijon mustard and half the lemon juice. Add the chicken to the marinade and set aside for about 30 minutes.

Add the zucchini and broccoli/broccolini to a bowl. Coat with the remaining olive oil, crushed garlic cloves and remaining lemon juice. Season with salt and pepper.

Add the chicken breast to a lined baking tray and cook for 10 minutes. Then add the broccoli and zucchini to the baking tray and roast for a further 10-15 minutes or until the chicken is cooked. Allow to rest for 5 minutes.

Build the bowl by adding the quinoa and topping with chicken, broccoli, zucchini, snow peas, avocado and pumpkin seeds.

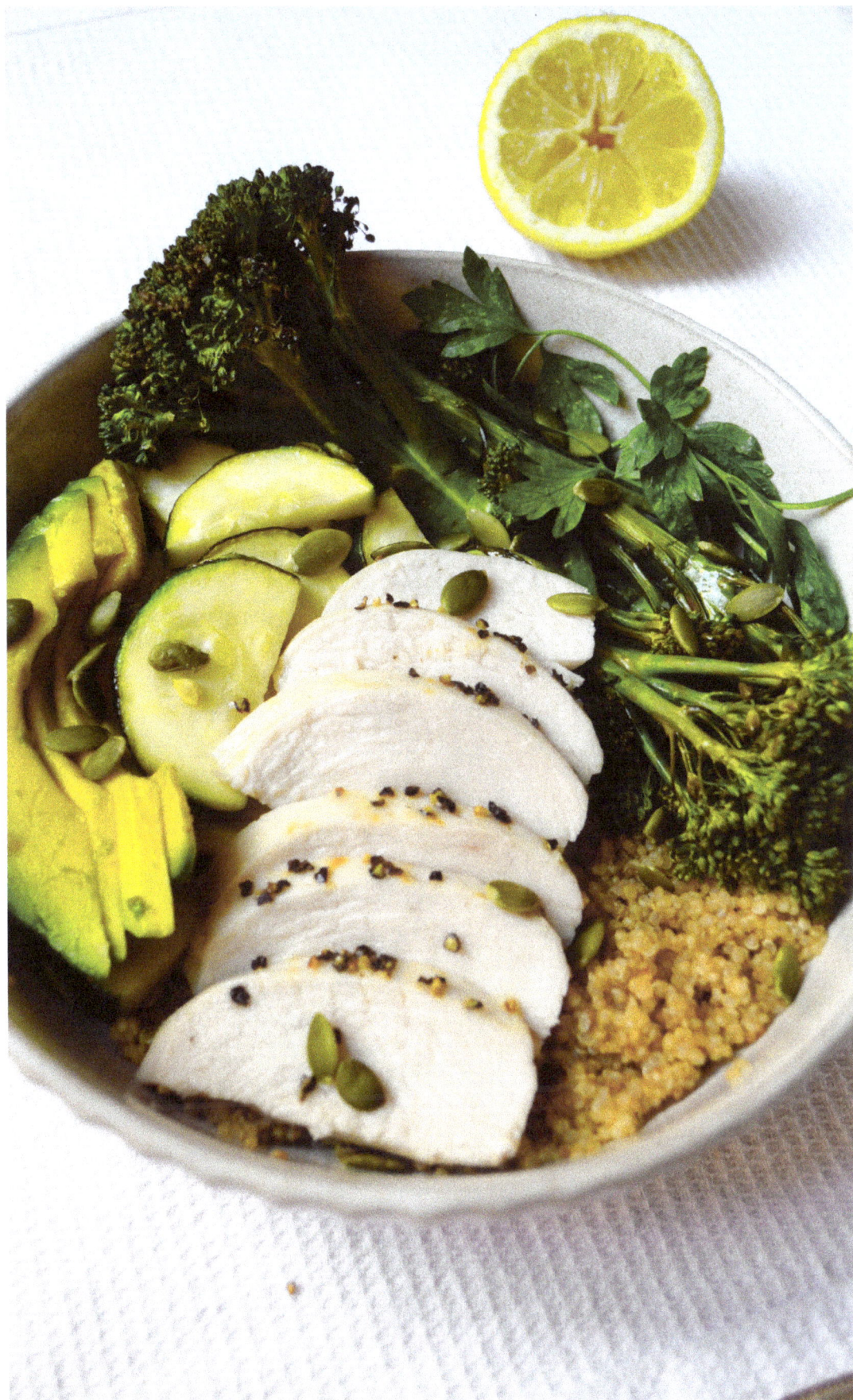

# CHICKEN NOODLE & VEGETABLE SOUP

**Serves:** 4    **Prep:** 15 minutes    **Cook:** 50 minutes

½ tbsp olive oil
500g chicken thighs/
  breast*
1 white onion, diced
2 garlic cloves, chopped
¼ bunch parsley, stems and
  leaves separated and
  finely chopped
2 carrots, halved and sliced
1 cup frozen peas
3 tbsp dried thyme
4 cups chicken stock or
  bone broth (see page 245)
3 cups water
400g corn kernels, drained
  and rinsed
½ cup string beans, cut into
  thirds
1 cup short angel hair pasta
2 cups spinach
2 zucchinis, halved and
  sliced
1 broccolini bunch, chopped
  into 3cm pieces/quartered
Salt and pepper to taste
1 lemon, juiced (optional)

In a large heated pot with olive oil, add the chicken and brown on both sides for 7-10 minutes. Remove from the pan and set aside.

In the same pan add the onion, garlic and parsley stems. Sauté for 3-5 minutes. Add the carrots and continue to cook for 10 minutes. Add the peas and thyme and continue to cook for 2 minutes.

Add the chicken stock, water, corn and string beans and bring to the boil. Reduce to simmer and cook until vegetables are almost tender. Then add the pasta to the soup and cook.

In the last 2 minutes of the pasta cooking, add the spinach, zucchini, broccolini and chopped parsley leaves and cook until just tender. Season with salt and pepper and add the juice of the lemon if using.

Before serving, shred or chop the chicken thighs/breasts, depending on your preference.

Serve the soup into bowls and evenly distribute the chicken across the servings.

**NOTE:**
› If you are short on time, you can use roast chicken and shred the meat.

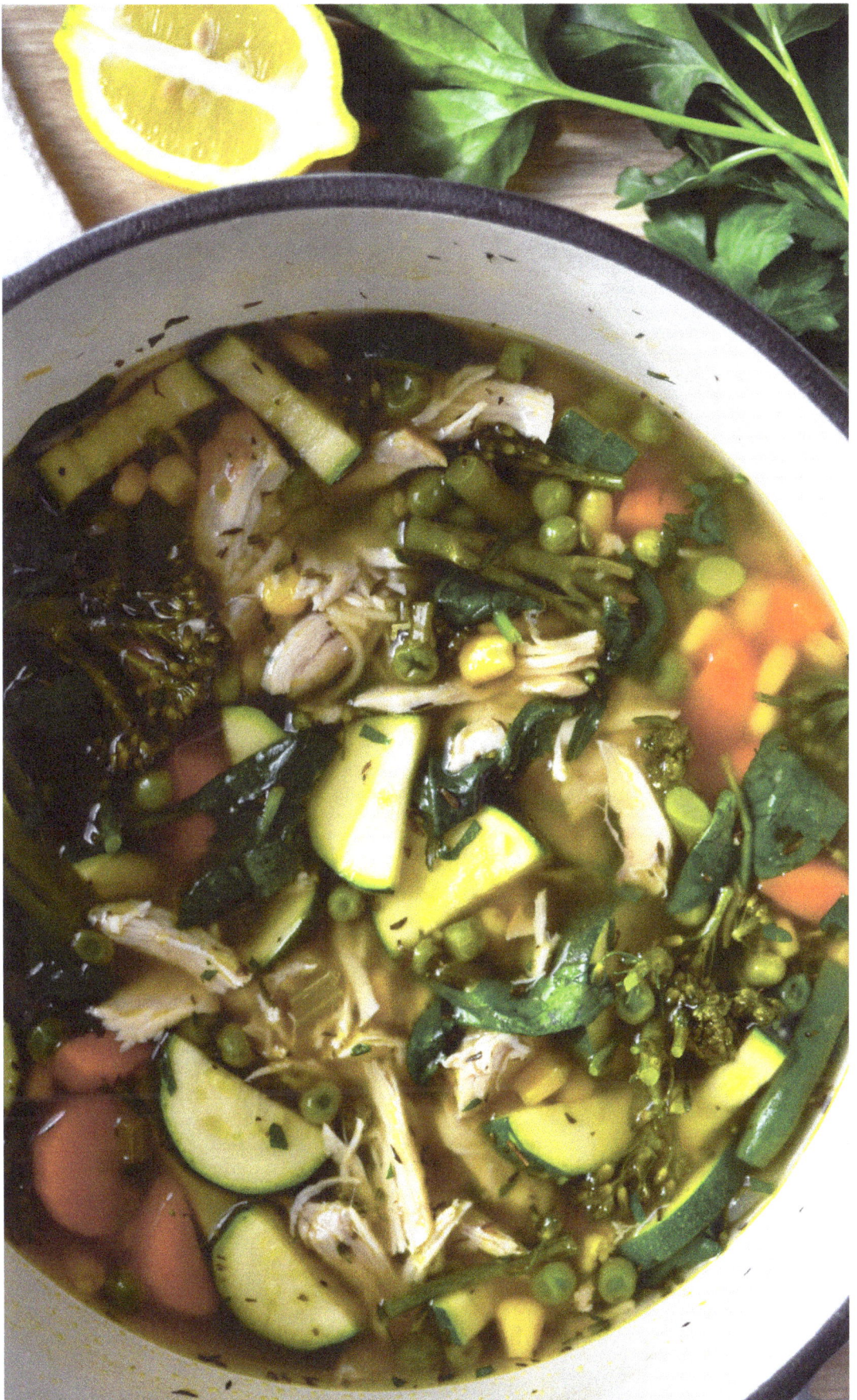

# FOLLICULAR PHASE BUDDHA BOWL

**Serves:** 4     **Prep:** 10 minutes     **Cook:** 15 minutes

**For the bowl:**
1 zucchini, sliced
1 head of broccoli, cut into
  florets
2 carrots, sliced
150g snow peas, ends
  trimmed
800g cannellini beans,
  drained and rinsed
2 garlic cloves, crushed
½ lemon, juiced
¼ cup parsley, chopped
2 cups quinoa, cooked
2 avocados
200g sprouts (crunchy or
  alfalfa)
4 tbsp hemp seeds

**For the dressing:**
¼ cup tahini
1 tbsp Dijon mustard
1 tsp turmeric
1 tbsp white wine vinegar
½ lemon, juiced

In a steamer or steaming basket over a pot of boiling water, steam the zucchini, broccoli, carrots and snow peas to your preference.

In a saucepan on medium heat, add the cannellini beans, garlic, lemon juice and parsley and cook for 2-3 minutes until slightly softened.

In a food processor, combine the tahini, Dijon, turmeric, white vinegar and lemon juice until a smooth consistency has formed.

Build the bowl by placing the quinoa at the base, followed by the vegetables, beans mix and avocado. Top with alfalfa sprouts, hemp seeds and a drizzle of dressing.

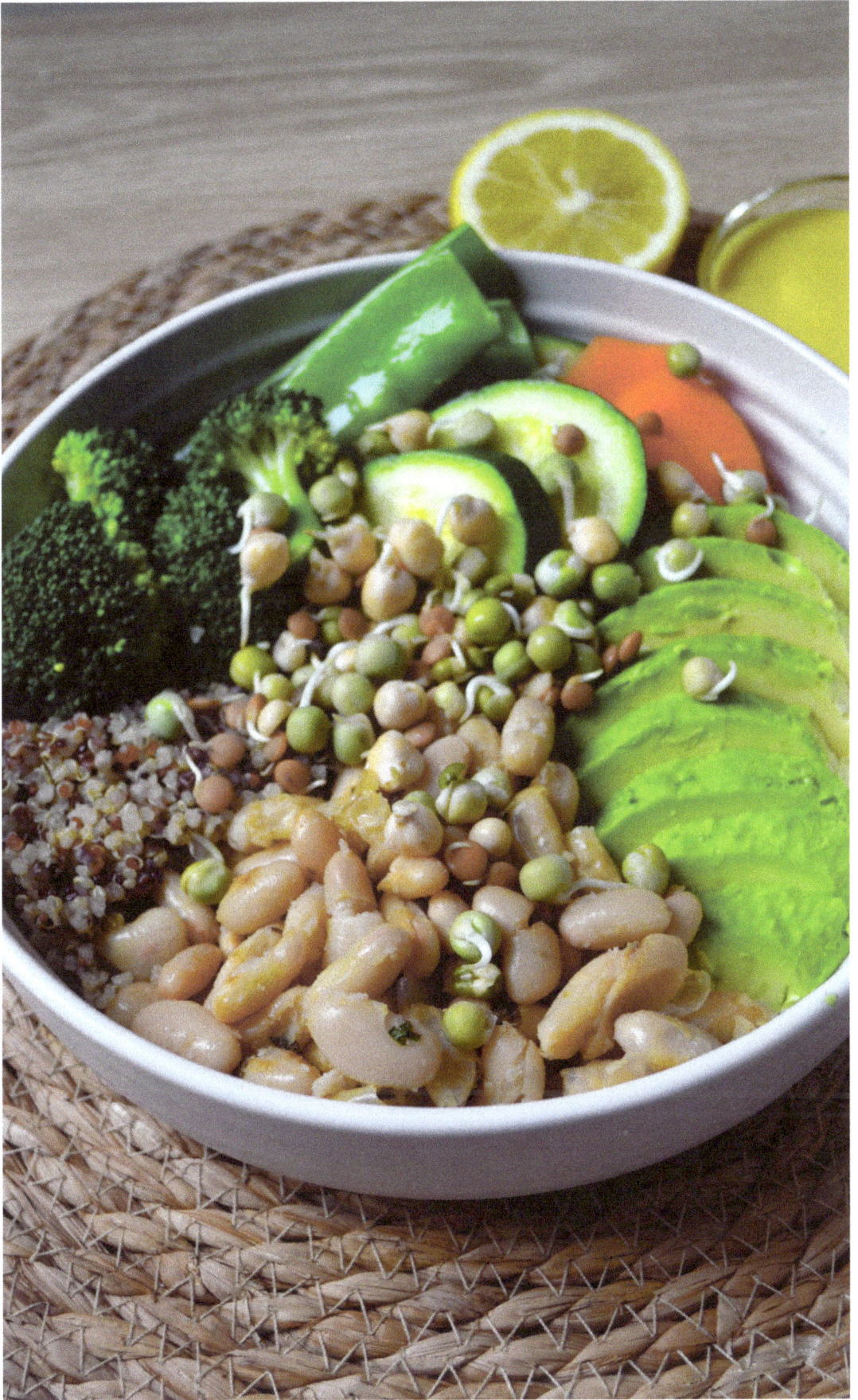

# CHICKEN PESTO PASTA

**Serves:** 2    **Prep:** 10 minutes    **Cook:** 20 minutes

**For the parsley pesto:**
1 cup parsley leaves, tightly packed*
2 cloves of garlic
1 tbsp lemon juice
2 tbsp pepita seeds
2 tbsp cashews (or sunflower seeds for a nut-free option)
1 tbsp nutritional yeast/parmesan
¼ cup olive oil
Salt to season, if desired

**For the pasta:**
Olive oil
1 onion, diced
2 garlic cloves, crushed
5 button mushrooms, sliced
1 chicken breast (approx 300g), diced
250g red lentil pasta
1 small zucchini, diced
½ cup frozen peas
1 cup spinach, roughly chopped
½ avocado, diced
Salt and pepper
1 spring onion, finely sliced

**To serve (optional):**
Parmesan
Spring onion, finely sliced
Fresh parsley or basil leaves

In a food processor, add all the ingredients for the parsley pesto. Blend until you get the consistency (chunky or fine) you desire. Set aside.*

In a frying pan on medium heat with a drizzle of olive oil, add the diced onion and chopped garlic. Sauté for 3-5 minutes.

Add the sliced mushrooms to the pan and cook for about 5 minutes until they have softened. Then add the diced chicken and cook until it is fully cooked through.

Meanwhile, cook the pasta according to the packet instructions.

Once the chicken is cooked through, add the zucchini and peas to the pan and cook for about 5 minutes until the zucchini is soft. Add the spinach and cook until it has wilted. Create a well in the center of the pan and add 2 tablespoons of pesto. Stir through evenly. Then add the diced avocado.

Drain the cooked pasta. Season with salt and pepper, a drizzle of olive oil and an additional tablespoon of pesto. Stir through and add more pesto if desired.

Serve the pasta with grated parmesan cheese, freshly chopped spring onion and fresh basil or parsley for added flavour if desired.

**NOTES:**
› You can opt for store bought basil pesto or use basil instead of parsley.
› Any leftover pesto can be stored in a jar, topped with olive oil and placed in the fridge for up to 2 weeks or frozen in ice cube trays.

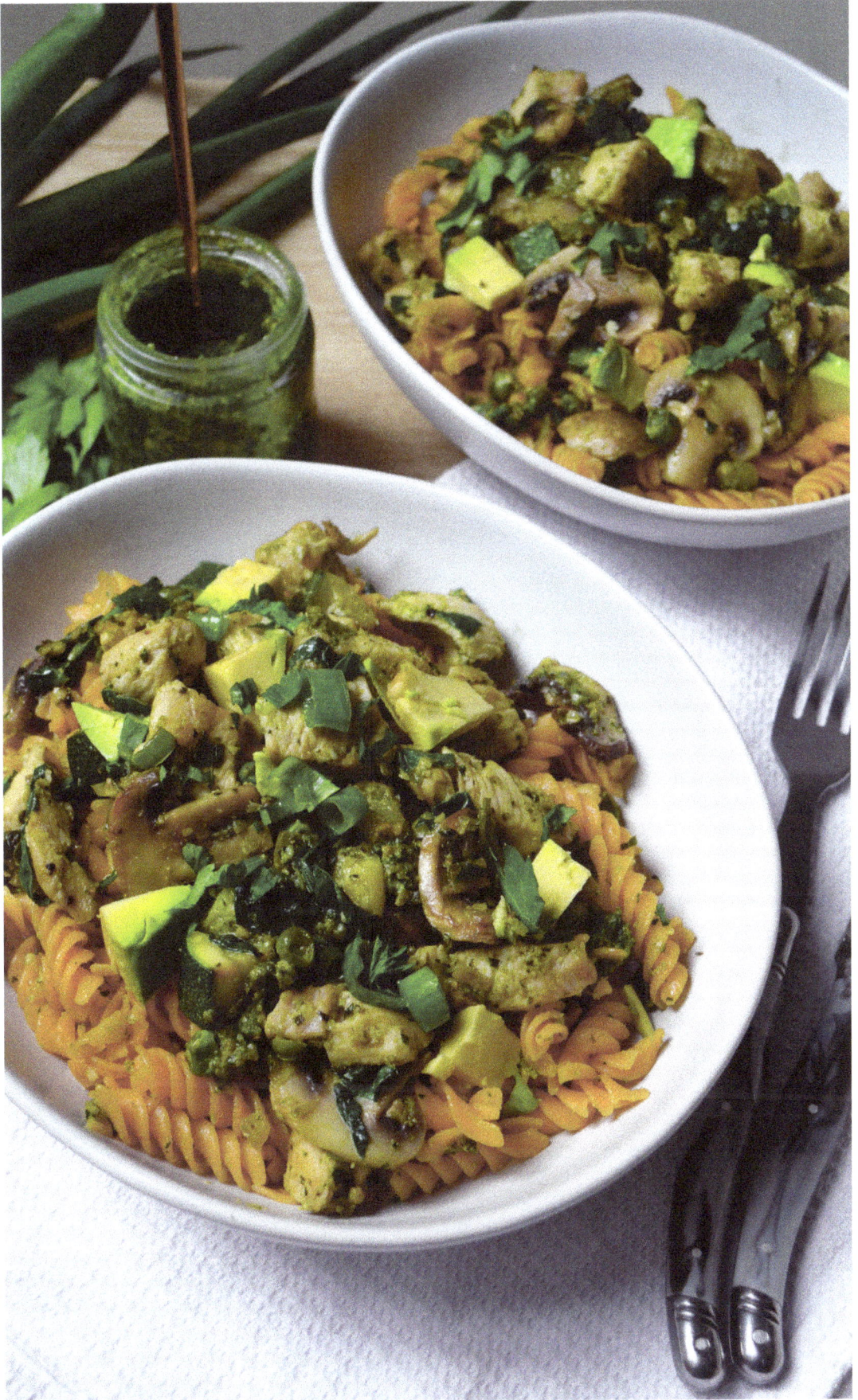

# SPRINGTIME STIRFRY

**Serves:** 4     **Prep:** 15 minutes     **Cook:** 20 minutes

2 chicken breasts, diced
2 tbsp whole grain mustard
1 tbsp olive oil
1 spring onion bunch,
   chopped into 8cm pieces
1 broccolini bunch, chopped
   into quarters
100g snow peas, ends
   trimmed
2 pak/bok choy bunches,
   sliced in half lengthways
3 garlic cloves, sliced
1 tbsp ginger, grated
1 red chilli (optional)
2 tbsp raw honey
1 lime, juiced
1 tbsp water

To serve:
Sesame seeds
Dried chilli flakes
Brown rice

Add the diced chicken, wholegrain mustard and olive oil into a bowl, stir through, and leave to marinate while preparing the vegetables.

Heat a frypan on medium with a little olive oil and add the chicken. Cook for 5-7 minutes until the chicken is cooked and then remove from pan.

Add the spring onion, broccolini and snow peas to the pan and cook for 2-3 minutes. Add the pak/bok choy, garlic, ginger and chilli and continue to cook until the vegetables are slightly tender but still crisp. Return the chicken to the pan.

Add the honey, lime juice and water to the pan and stir through, coating all the chicken and vegetables.

Serve with a sprinkle of sesame seeds and dried chilli flakes, if desired. Serve on its own or with some brown rice.

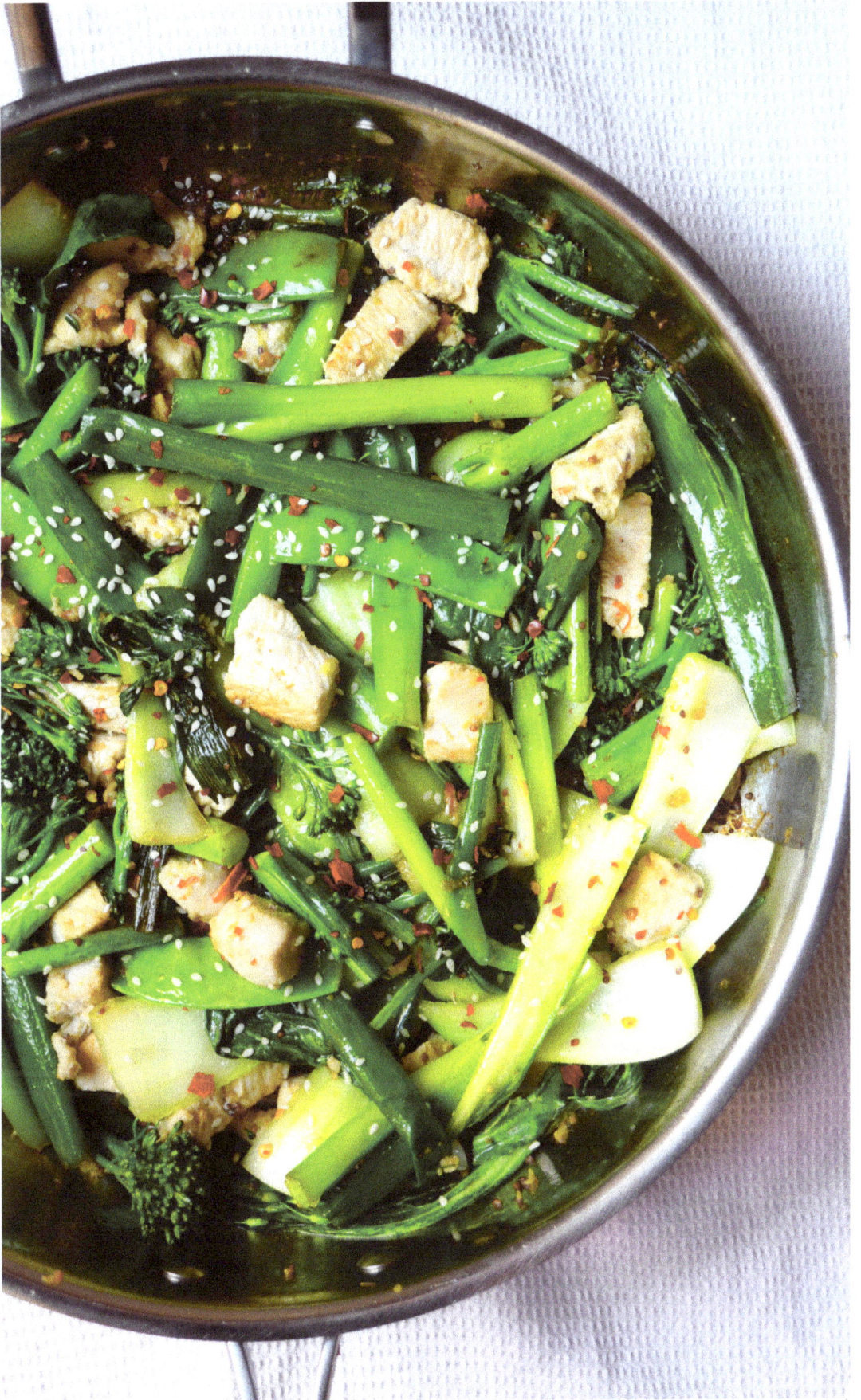

# POACHED CHICKEN
## WITH RAW VEGGIE SALAD &
## SATAY DRESSING

**Serves:** 4    **Prep:** 15 minutes    **Cook:** 30 minutes

2 chicken breasts
1 lemon, juiced
Salt and pepper
1 zucchini, grated
2 carrots, grated
1 capsicum, finely sliced
¼ red cabbage, finely
  shredded
½ bunch coriander,
  chopped
¼ bunch spring onions,
  finely sliced
1 cup snow peas, julienned
½ cup alfalfa sprouts
¼ cup raw cashews

For the satay dressing:
2 tbsp peanut butter
1 tbsp tamari/soy sauce
1 tbsp ginger, grated
1-2 limes, juiced
1 tbsp sweet chilli sauce
¼-½ cup water

To serve:
Coriander leaves
Chilli (fresh or flakes)
Cashews, roughly chopped

Remove the chicken breasts from the fridge and allow them to sit at room temperature for 30 minutes. Then bring a pot of water to boil and add the lemon, salt and pepper to the water. Add the chicken breasts and cover, building it back to a boil. Once boiled, removed from the heat and allow the chicken to poach in the hot water for 20 minutes.

In a bowl, combine the zucchini, carrots, capsicum, cabbage, coriander, spring onions, snow peas, alfalfa sprouts and cashews.

Make the satay sauce by combining the peanut butter, tamari/soy sauce, ginger, lime juice and sweet chilli sauce in a bowl. Use a stick blender to combine well. Add water gradually to create a thinner consistency.

Once the chicken is cooked, remove it from the water and either slice or shred. Add to the salad.

Dress the salad with the satay dressing, toss well to combine and garnish with extra coriander, chilli and cashews to serve.

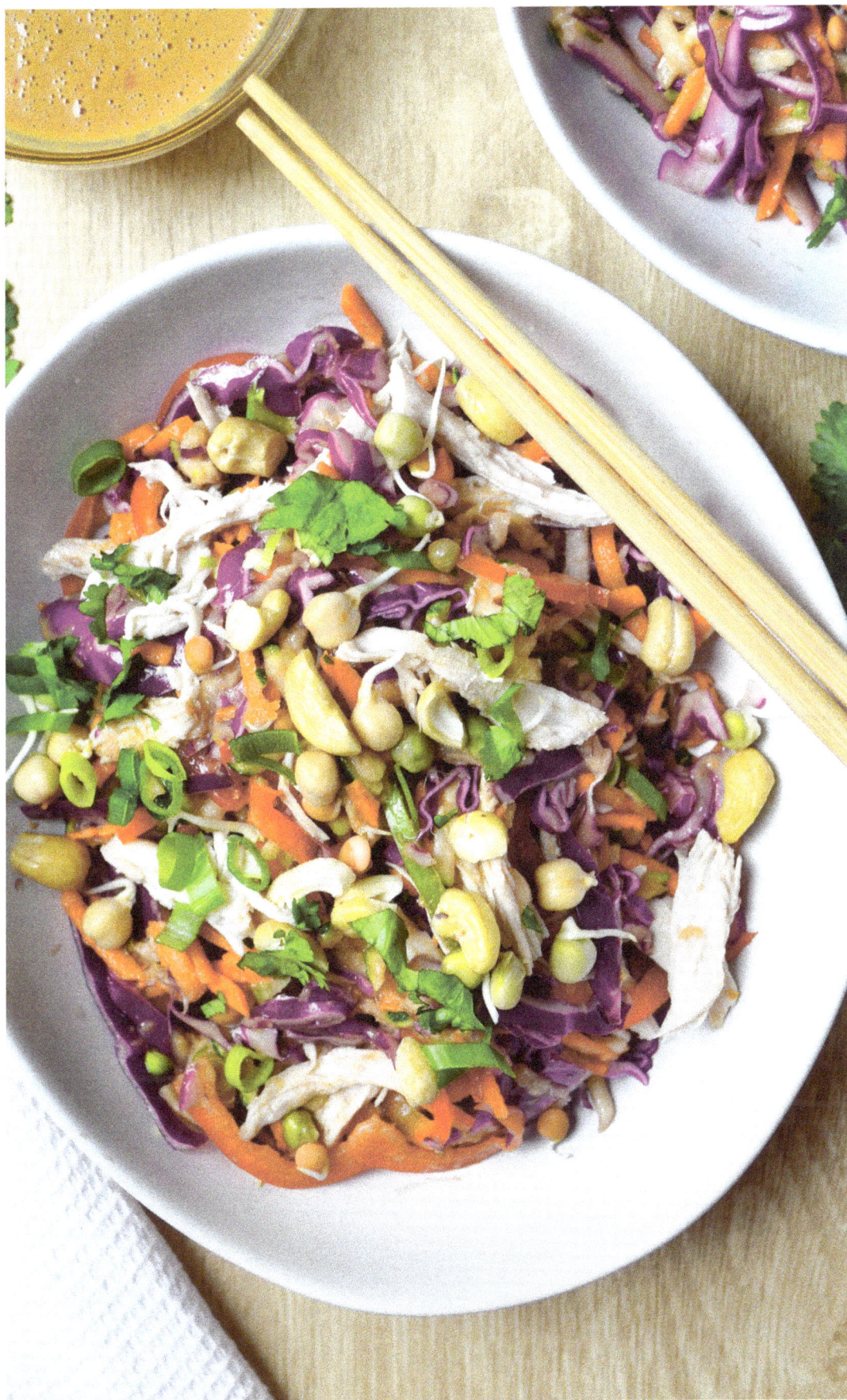

# NOURISH PLATES

**Serves:** 4     **Prep:** 10 minutes     **Cook:** 25 minutes

4 chicken sausages (or protein of choice)
2 cups corn kernels
4 boiled eggs
4 cans tuna, drained
½ cup sauerkraut or kimchi
2 cucumbers, sliced into sticks
2 carrots, sliced into sticks
1 celery stick, sliced into sticks (optional)
1 punnet cherry tomatoes
½ cup olives
½ cup baby pickled cucumbers
4 square cheese slices
Dip of choice
Olive oil
Salt and pepper

Preheat the oven to 180°C fan-forced.

On a lined baking tray, add the sausages and place in the oven for about 20 minutes or until cooked. On another lined baking dish, add the corn kernels. Drizzle with olive oil and season with salt and pepper. Bake for 10-15 minutes or until lightly roasted.

Once the sausages and corn have been cooked, construct your plate by equally dividing all the ingredients across the 4 plates or containers. Adjust the portions to your preference.

**NOTE:**
› The nourish plates make for a great and easy meal that will support hormones across the cycle. You can substitute items according to the different hero ingredients to adapt it to different phases of the cycle. Fermented and pickled foods are great in the follicular phase as well as good for overall gut health, which is essential for good hormone health.

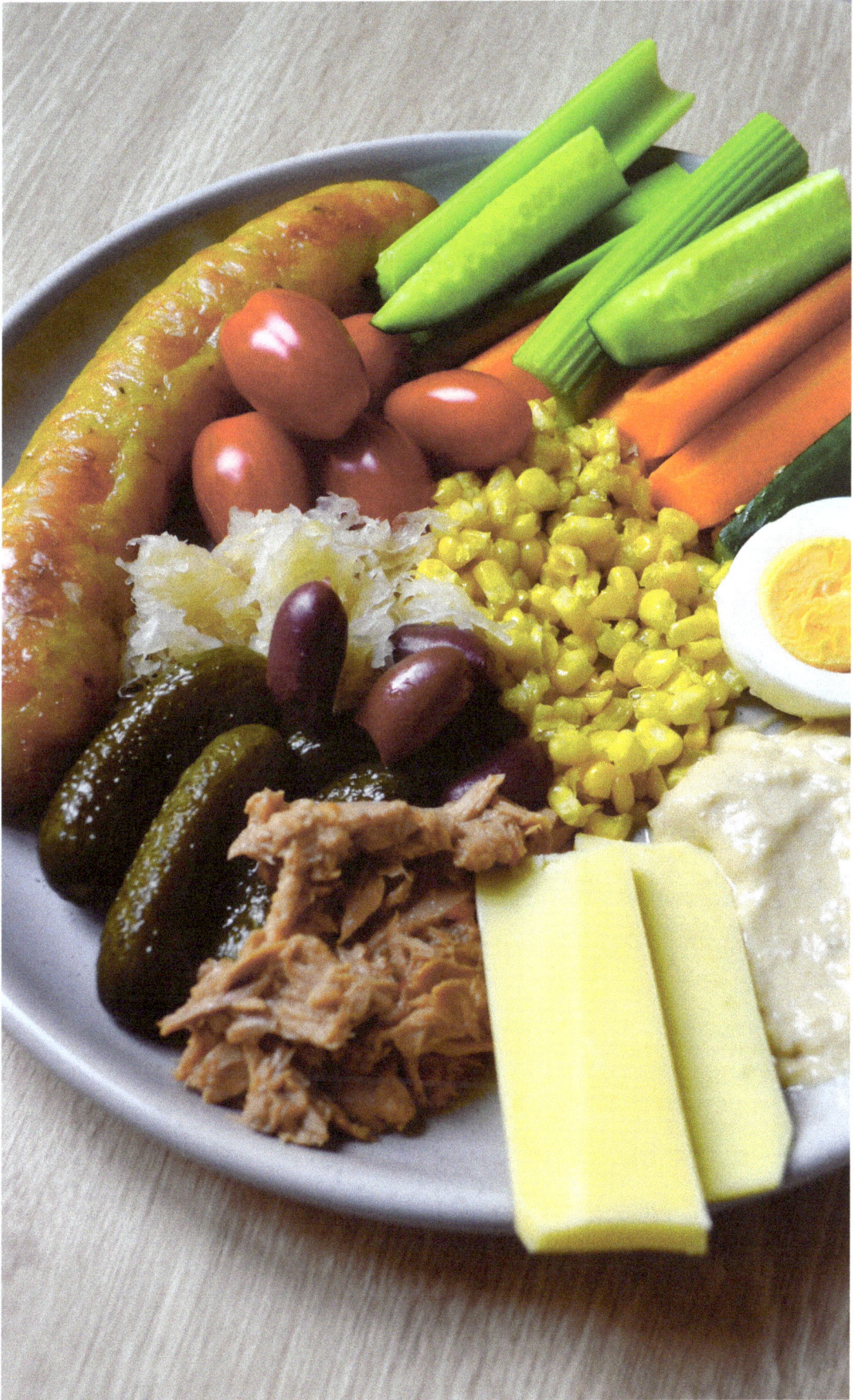

# GREEK NOURISH BOWLS

**Serves:** 4     **Prep:** 15 minutes     **Cook:** 20 minutes

**For the chicken:**
4 chicken breasts, diced
1 garlic clove, minced
1 tbsp olive oil
1 lemon, juiced
1 tbsp oregano
Salt and pepper

**For the quinoa:**
1 cup quinoa
2 ½ cups water
1 tbsp olive oil
1 tbsp red wine vinegar

**For the tzatziki dip:**
1 cup Greek yoghurt
1 garlic clove
½ lemon, juiced
½ cucumber, grated
1 tbsp fresh dill, chopped

**For the bowl:**
2 cucumbers, sliced
1 punnet cherry tomatoes,
  halved
⅓ cup kalamata olives,
  halved
150g feta, crumbled
  (optional)
Fresh dill, chopped
  (optional)

Preheat the oven to 180°C fan-forced.

In a bowl, combine the diced chicken, garlic, olive oil, lemon juice, oregano and salt and pepper. Transfer to a lined baking tray and bake in the oven for 15-20 minutes or until the chicken is cooked through.

Meanwhile, add the quinoa and water into a pot. Cover and bring to boil. Remove the lid and reduce to a simmer, stirring regularly. Cook until the water has evaporated and the quinoa has cooked. Remove from the heat and dress with olive oil and red wine vinegar. Set aside.

To make the tzatziki, combine the yoghurt, garlic, lemon, cucumber and dill. Set aside.

Build the bowls by equally dividing the ingredients. Start by adding the quinoa, then top with chicken, cucumber, tomatoes, olives, feta (if using) and the tzatziki dip. Garnish with dill if using.

**NOTE:**
› Substitute the chicken for lamb and this recipe doubles as an ovulatory phase recipe too.

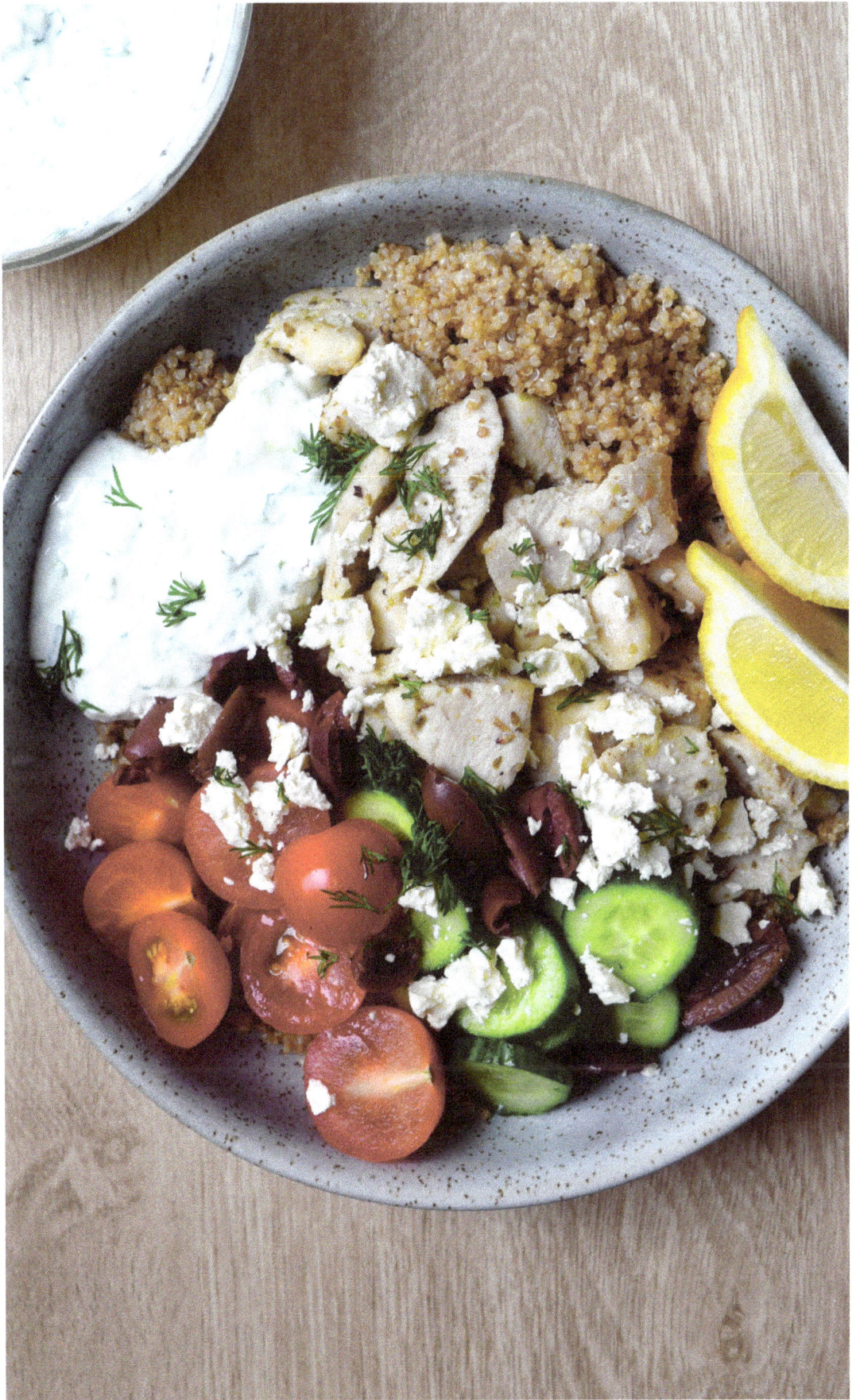

# LENTIL & PARSLEY SALAD

**Serves:** 4     **Prep:** 15 minutes     **Cook:** 10 minutes

½ cup quinoa
1 ½ cups water
800g canned lentils,
    drained and rinsed
1 parsley bunch, chopped
2 cups spinach, chopped
¼ cup pepitas
½ cup sunflower seeds
¼ cup dried cranberries,
    chopped
2 tbsp capers
1 red onion, finely diced
1 tbsp olive oil
½ lemon, juiced

**For the yoghurt dressing:**
1 cup Greek yoghurt
1 tsp cumin
½ lemon, juiced
1 tsp honey

Add the quinoa and water to a pot on medium-high heat. Cover with a lid and bring it to a boil. Remove lid and reduce to a simmer, stirring regularly. Cook until the water has evaporated and the quinoa has cooked. Remove from heat and set aside.

In a bowl, combine the lentils, parsley, spinach, pepitas, sunflower seeds, cranberries, capers, onion and cooked quinoa. Drizzle with olive oil and lemon juice. Season with salt and pepper if desired.

To make the dressing, mix the yoghurt, cumin, lemon juice and honey in a separate bowl.

Top the salad with the yoghurt dressing when ready to serve.

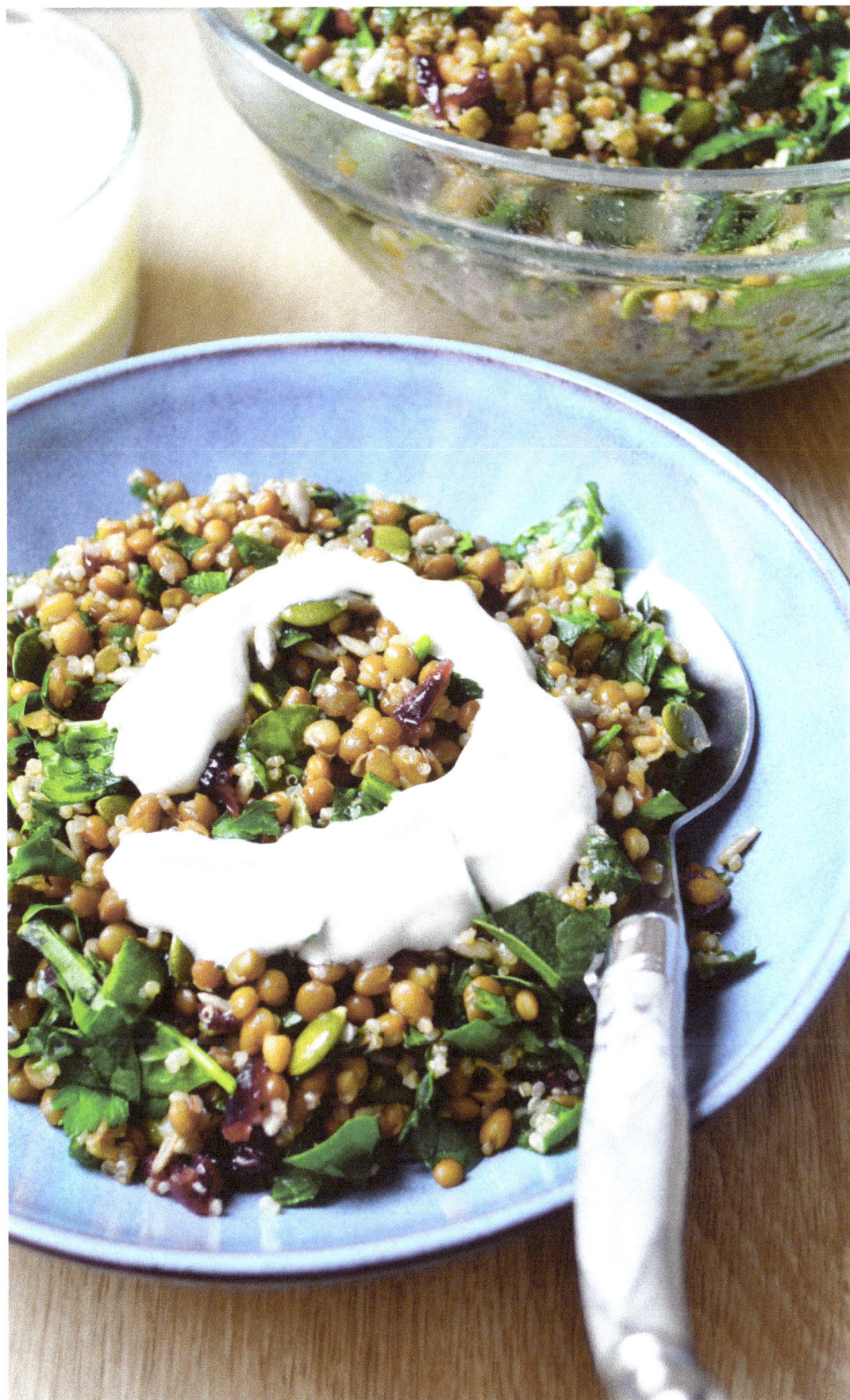

# LEMON PEPPER CHICKEN
## WITH MASHED PEAS &
## SUNDRIED TOMATO SAUCE

**Serves:** 2      **Prep:** 10 minutes      **Cook:** 45 minutes

**For the chicken:**
2 chicken breasts
½ tsp olive oil
1 tsp lemon pepper
  seasoning

**For the steamed veggies:**
1 small broccoli head, cut
  into florets
1 small zucchini, halved and
  cut lengthways
1 carrot, peeled and diced
Salt and pepper to season

**For the pea mash:**
1 cup frozen green peas
½ cup water
1 lemon, juiced
1 garlic clove

**For the sauce:**
1 capsicum, halved
¼ cup sundried tomatoes
1 tsp smoked paprika
½ avocado
⅓ cup water (add more for a
  thinner consistency)

Preheat the oven to 180°C fan-forced and line a baking tray.

Place the chicken breasts on the tray and cover in olive oil and lemon pepper seasoning. On the same tray, add the capsicum with a drizzle of olive oil. Bake in the oven for 25-30 minutes or until the chicken is cooked through.

Meanwhile, add the broccoli and zucchini to a steaming basket above a pot of boiling water. Cover the basket with a lid and steam for 3 minutes until slightly tender and bright green. Remove from the basket and set aside.

Now add the carrot to the steaming basket, cover with a lid and steam for about 5 minutes or until the carrots are tender to your liking. Remove from the basket and set aside with the broccoli and zucchini. Season all with salt and pepper.

Put the frozen peas and water in a microwave-safe bowl and microwave for 2 minutes. Drain the remaining water and add the lemon juice and garlic. Using a stick blender, blend the mash until it forms a pureed texture and then set aside.

Once the chicken is cooked through, remove the tray from the oven and allow to rest while making the capsicum sauce.

In a bowl or jug, add the capsicum, sundried tomatoes, smoked paprika, avocado and water and blend until smooth. Adjust the flavours and texture with more smoked paprika or water if desired.

Serve the chicken and steamed veggies on a bed of mashed peas and top with the capsicum and sundried tomato sauce.

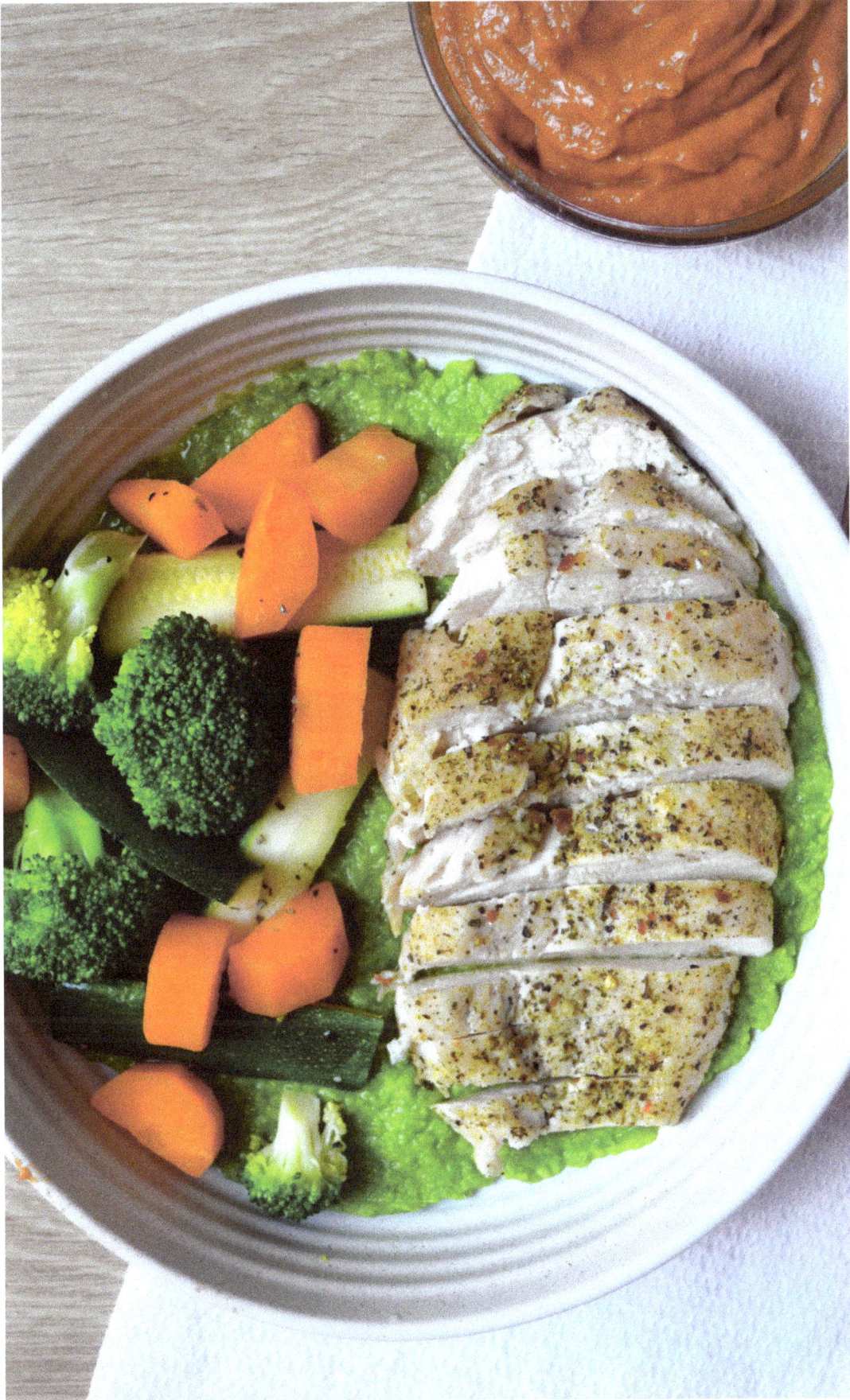

# snacks

Plum Slice

Banana Oat
Biscuits

Trail Bites

Coconut
Lemon Slice

Smoky Carrot Dip

Carrot Cake
Bliss Balls

# PLUM SLICE

**Serves:** 8     **Prep:** 5 minutes     **Cook:** 40 minutes

**For the base:**
1 cup oats
½ cup cashews
¼ cup sunflower seeds
⅓ cup coconut oil, melted

**For the plum layer:**
3-4 red plums
1 tsp water
1 tbsp orange or lemon juice
1 tsp cinnamon

**Optional toppings:**
Cashews, roughly chopped
Coconut flakes
Oats
Sunflower seeds
Pepitas

Preheat the oven to 180°C fan-forced.

In a food processor, blend the oats, cashews and sunflower seeds until a flour-like consistency has formed. Add the melted coconut oil and blend until crumbly.

In a lined bread tin, add the base mixture and press down until an even layer has been formed. Place in the oven for 15 minutes.

Roughly chop the plums and add to a saucepan with the water, orange or lemon juice and cinnamon. Cook for about 15 minutes or until they have begun to stew and reduce. Pour the plum mixture onto the base and garnish with toppings of choice.

Cook in the oven for a further 20 minutes.

Remove from the oven and allow to cool. Slice into squares.

Store in the fridge until ready to eat.

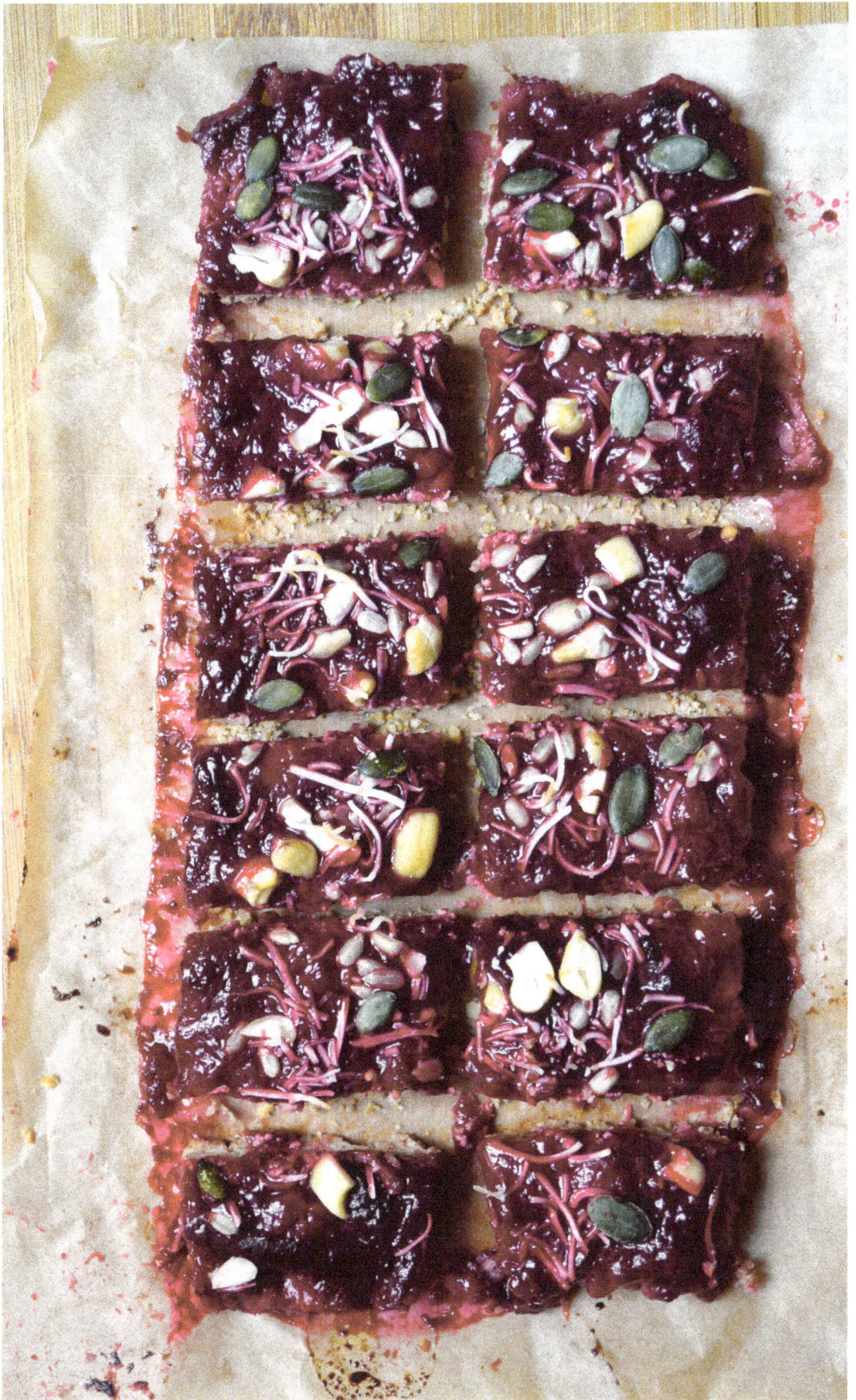

# BANANA OAT BISCUITS

**Serves:** 10-12     **Prep:** 10 minutes     **Cook:** 25 minutes

2 ripe bananas, mashed
3 tbsp peanut butter
1 tbsp flaxseed meal
½ cup water
1 tbsp chopped dates or
  maple syrup
2 cups oats
1 tsp cacao powder
¼ cup dark chocolate,
  chopped
Extra chocolate for drizzling
  (optional)

Preheat the oven to 180°C fan-forced.

In a mixing bowl, combine the banana, peanut butter, flaxseed meal, water and dates/maple syrup.

Stir in the oats, cacao powder and dark chocolate pieces.

Roll the mixture into balls and press into a biscuit shape, placing them onto a lined baking tray. Bake in the oven for 20-25 minutes until cooked.

If desired, melt some dark chocolate and drizzle it onto the cooked biscuits.

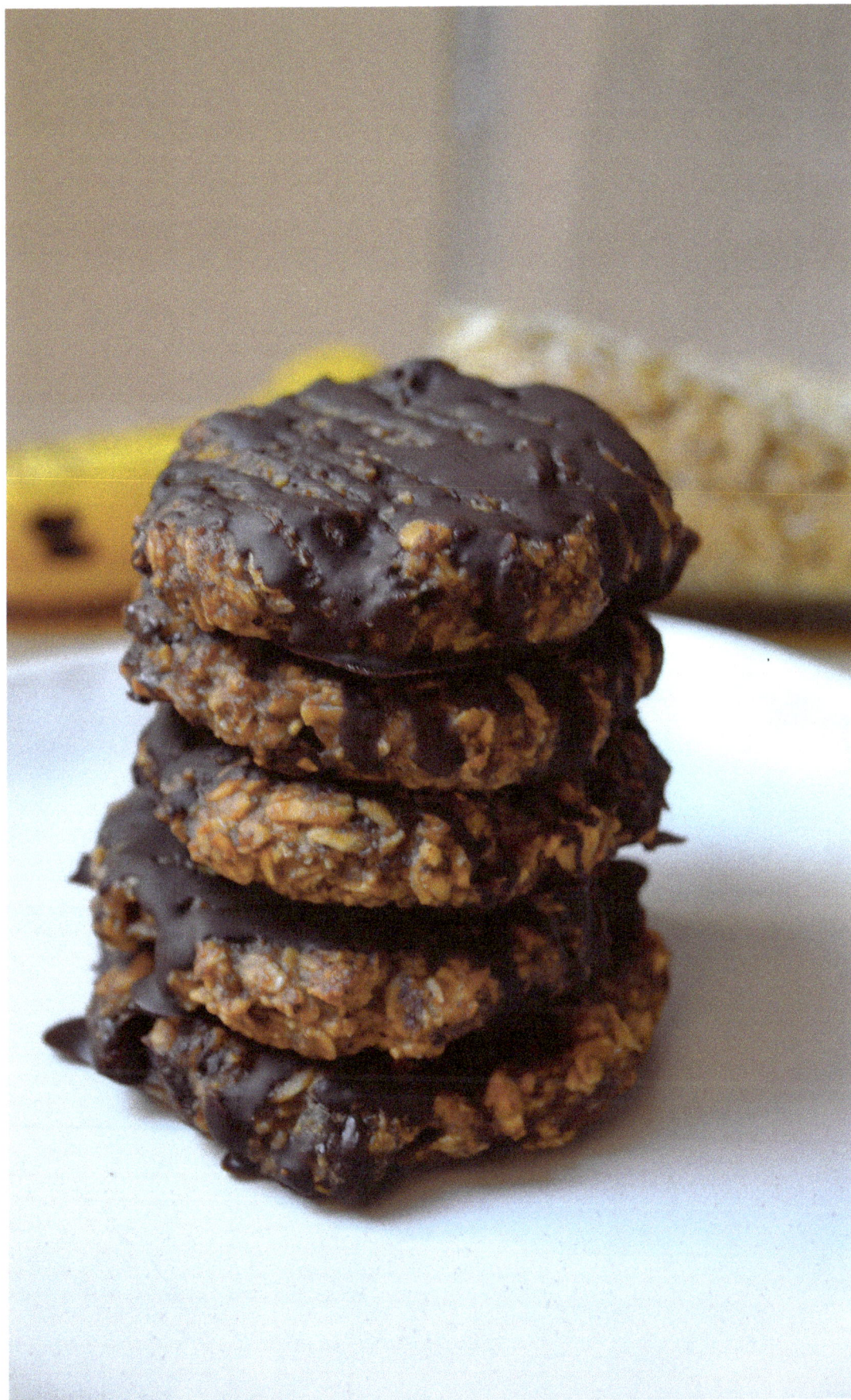

# TRAIL BITES

**Serves:** 12     **Prep:** 10 minutes     **Cook:** 30 minutes

½ cup brazil nuts
½ cup cashew nuts
¼ cup almonds
¼ cup pepitas
¼ cup sunflower seeds
1 tbsp sesame seeds
1 tbsp chia seeds
4 medjool dates, pitted
1 tbsp dried cranberries
½ tsp cinnamon
½ tsp nutmeg
1 tbsp nut butter
1 tbsp maple syrup
½ tsp vanilla extract
1 tbsp flaxseed meal
3 tbsp water

Preheat the oven to 140°C fan-forced.

In a food processor, add all the nuts, seeds, dates, cranberries, cinnamon and nutmeg. Blitz until nuts are coarsely chopped.

In a separate bowl, combine the nut butter, maple syrup, vanilla extract, flaxseed meal and water.

Mix the dry and wet ingredients together until well combined.

Using wet hands, roll the mixture into balls and place on a lined baking tray. Press down the balls to make biscuit-shaped pieces.

Bake in the oven for 25-30 minutes. Allow to cool before consuming.

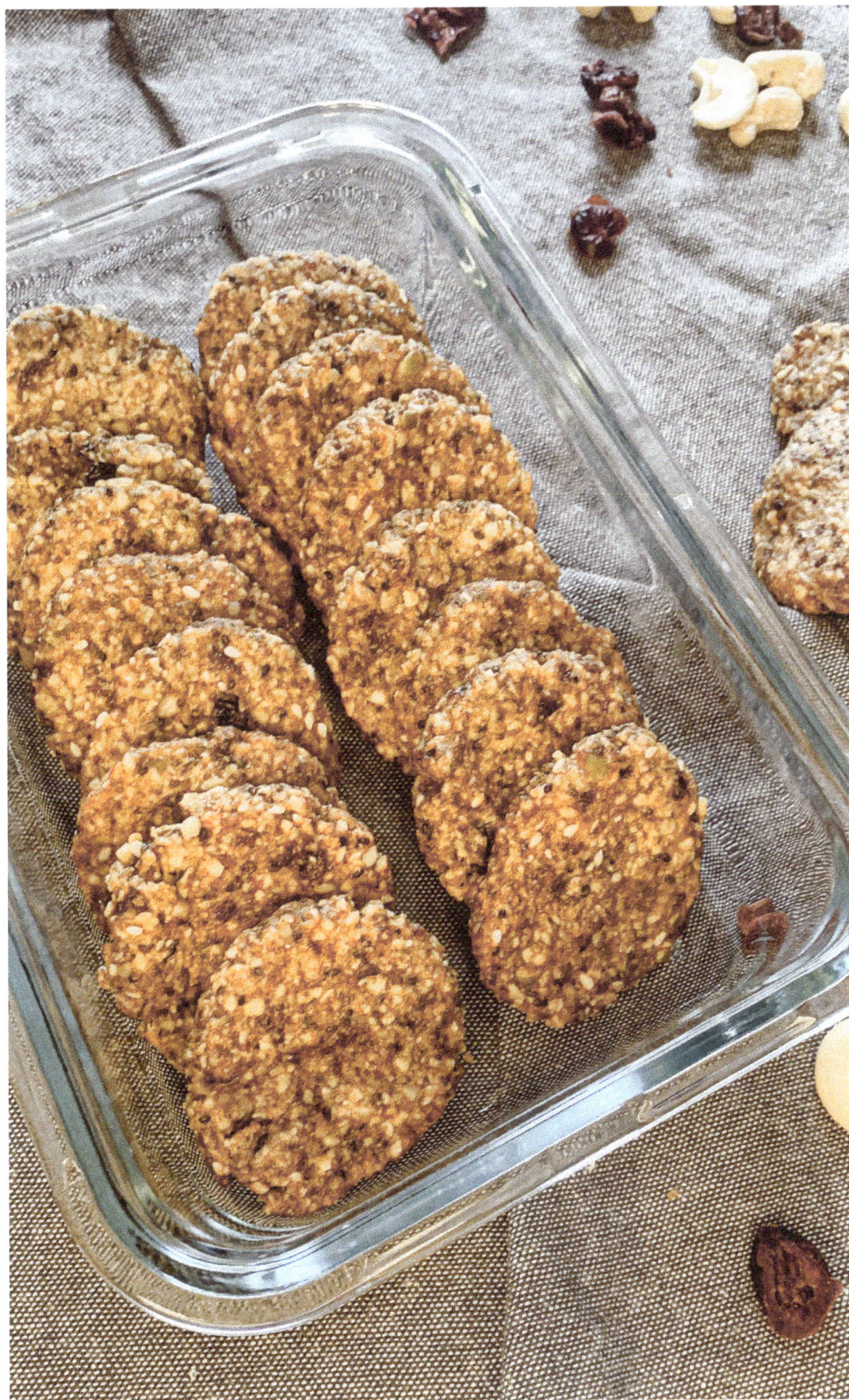

# COCONUT LEMON SLICE

**Serves:** 6       **Prep:** 10 minutes       **Cook:** 1hr 30 minutes+

**For the base:**
8 medjool dates
½ cup cashews
½ cup brazil nuts
½ cup desiccated coconut
¼ cup flaxseed meal
¼ cup pepitas
1 lemon, zested and juiced
¼ cup water

**For the topping:**
1 cup cashews
1 lemon, juiced
¼ cup desiccated coconut
½ cup coconut oil
1 tbsp maple syrup
¼ cup water (to loosen
    mixture if needed)

Soak the cashews for the topping in a bowl of water and set aside.

In a food processor, combine the dates, cashews, brazil nuts, coconut, flaxseed meal, pepitas, lemon zest and juice, and water. Blend until combined.

Transfer the base mixture into a bread tin and press down evenly. Refrigerate for 30 minutes to set.

Once the base has set, drain the cashews soaking in water. Add them and the lemon juice, coconut, coconut oil, maple syrup and water for the topping into a food processor or blender. Blend until a smooth creamy texture has formed. Add more water if the mixture is too thick.

Remove the base from the refrigerator and cover with the topping. Return to the fridge and allow to set for at least 1 hour.

Slice into bars or bites.

Store in an airtight container in the fridge for up to a week.

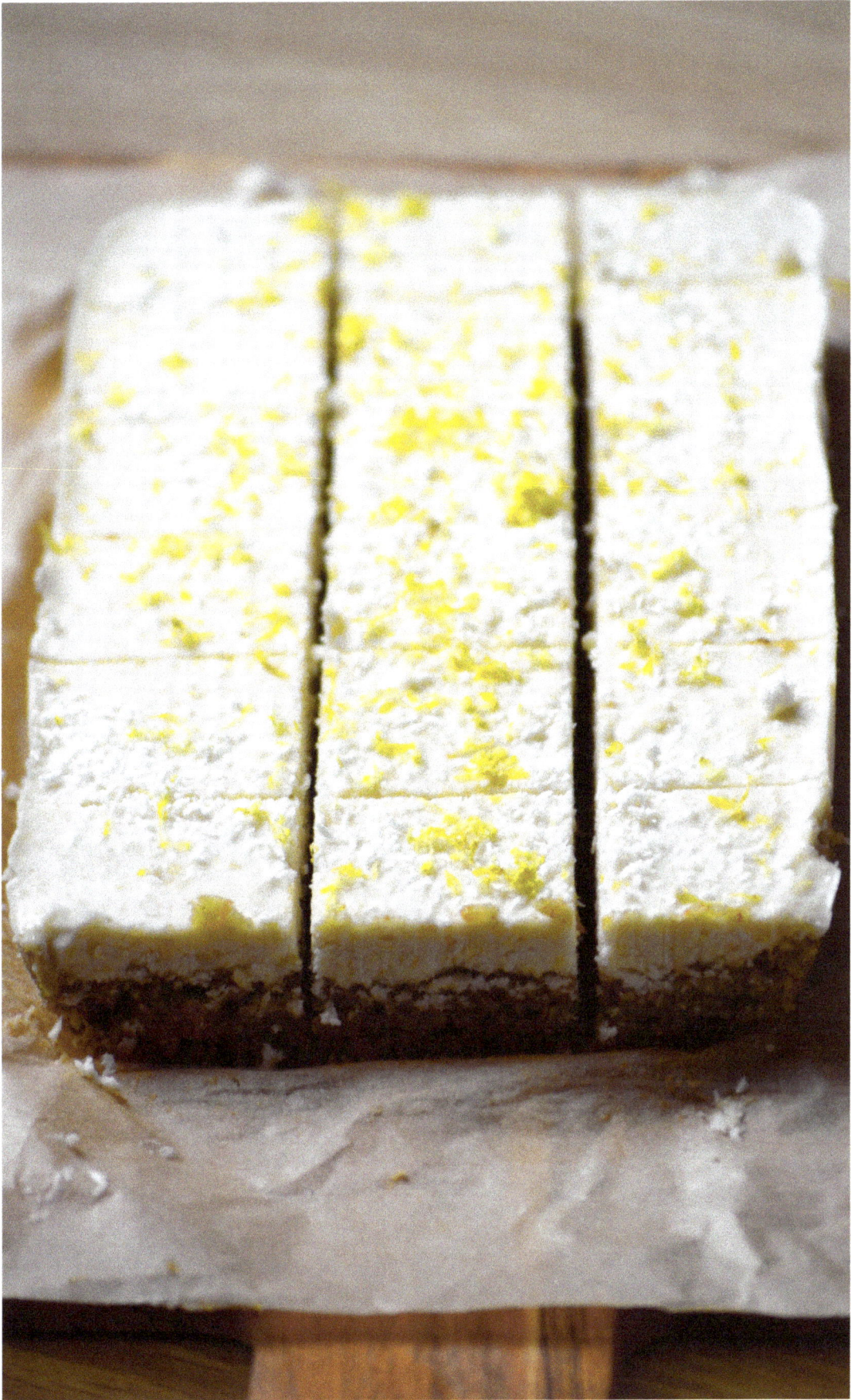

# SMOKY CARROT DIP

**Serves:** 1     **Prep:** 5 minutes     **Cook:** 30 minutes

4 carrots, peeled and
   quartered
Salt and pepper
Olive oil to drizzle
1 tsp smoked paprika
1 garlic clove
1 tbsp olive oil
1 tbsp water
1 lemon, juiced

Preheat the oven to 200°C fan-forced.

On a lined baking tray, add the carrots and season with salt and pepper and a drizzle of olive oil. Roast for 30 minutes. Remove from the oven and allow to cool slightly.

In a food processor, add the carrots, smoked paprika, garlic, olive oil, water and lemon juice. Blend until combined.

Enjoy with linseed crackers (see page 251) or fresh vegetable sticks.

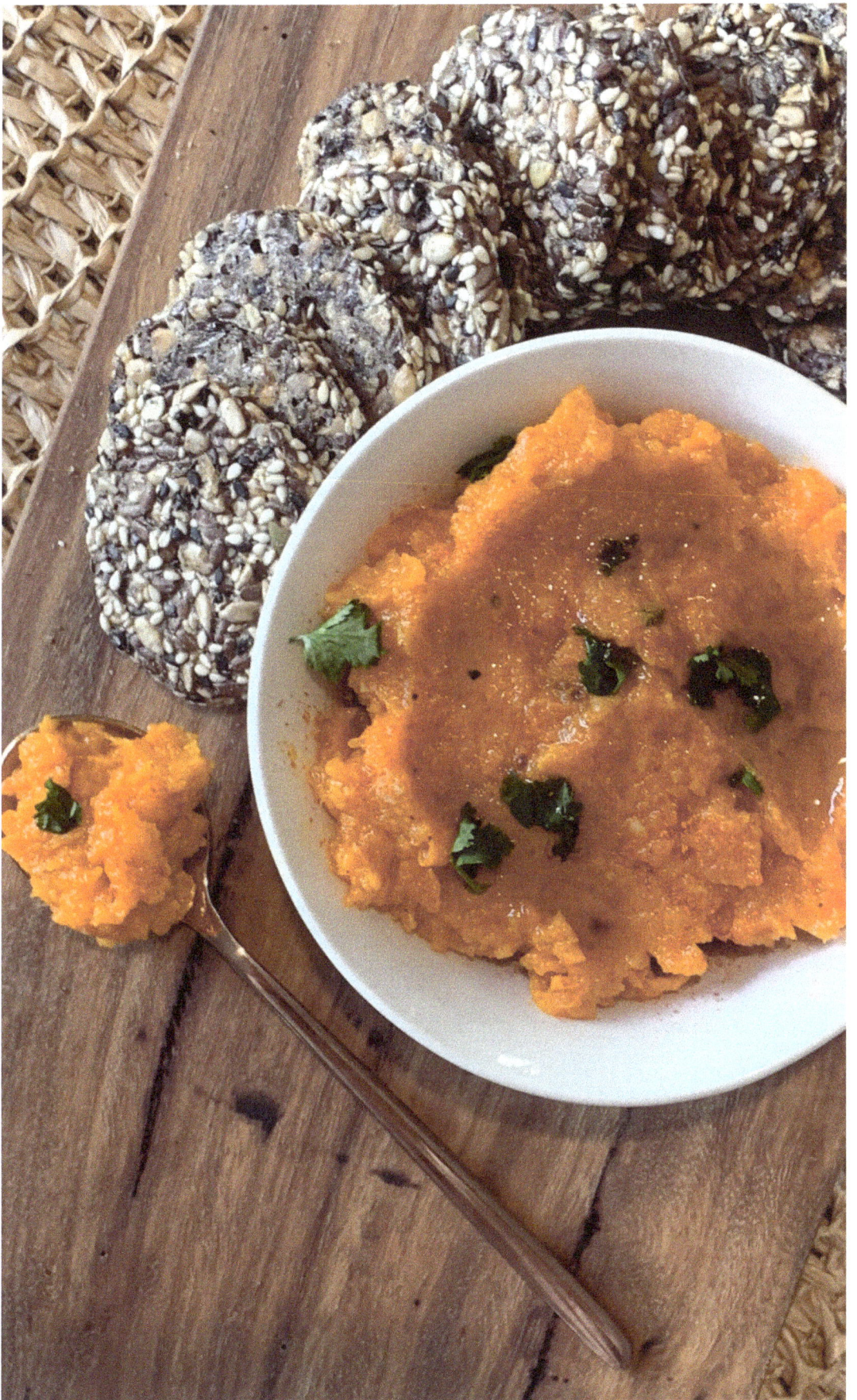

# CARROT CAKE BLISS BALLS

**Serves:** 8-12 balls   **Prep:** 10 minutes   **Cook:** 30 minutes

6 medjool dates
2 tbsp cashew butter
1 tbsp ginger, grated
1 tbsp maple syrup
1 tsp vanilla essence
¼ cup walnuts
1 tsp cinnamon
⅓ cup oats
½ cup grated carrot
¼ cup walnuts, crushed (for coating)

Add all the ingredients (except for the crushed walnuts for coating) into a food processor and blitz until combined.

With damp hands, roll the mixture into balls and set on a tray or plate. Refrigerate for 30 minutes to set.

If using, coat the carrot cake balls in crushed walnuts.

Store in an airtight container in the fridge for up to a week.

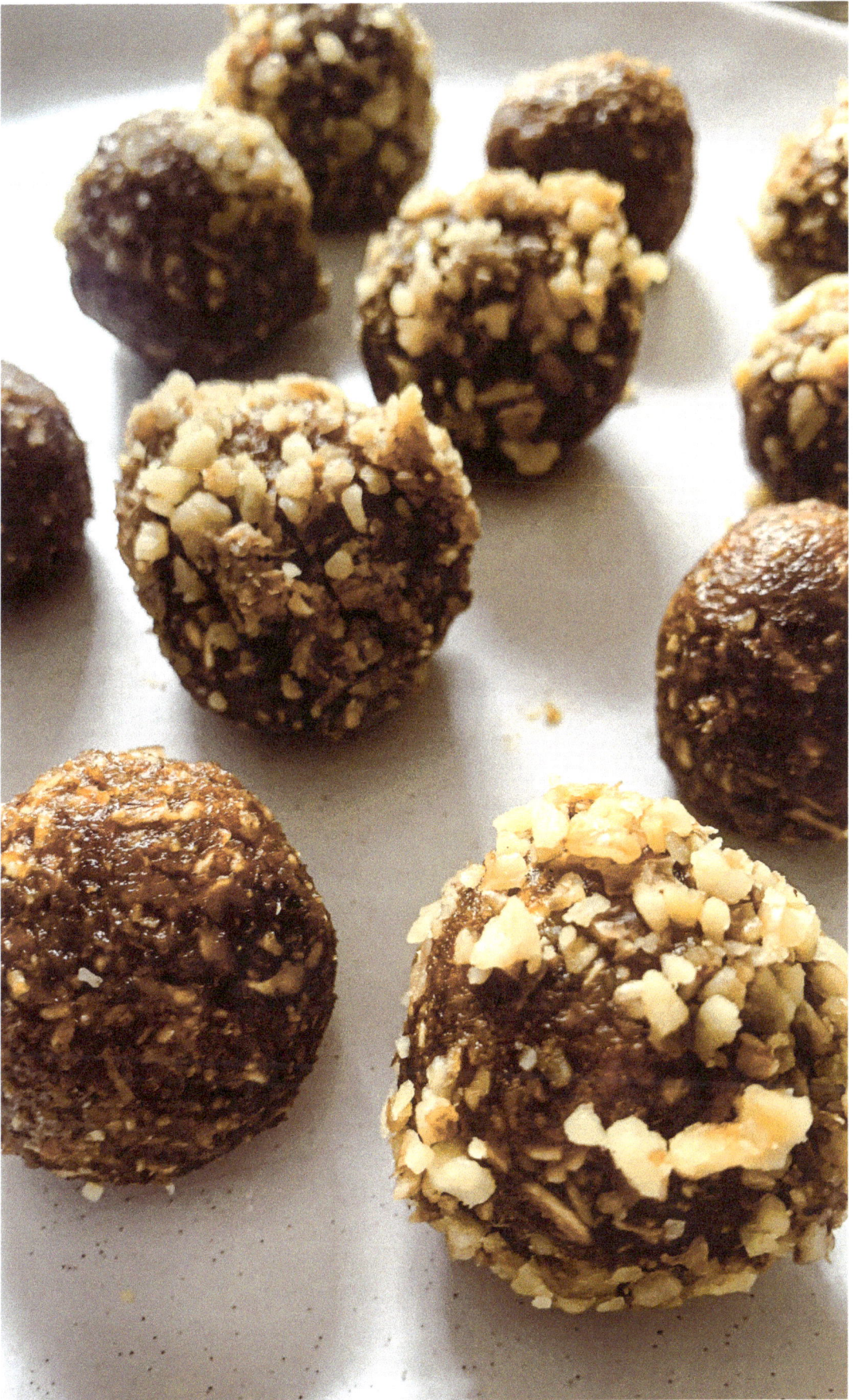

ovulatory phase

# HERO FOODS

**NUTRIENTS FOR THE OVULATORY PHASE**

ZINC | CALCIUM | OMEGA-3S | FIBRE

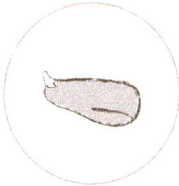

EGGPLANT

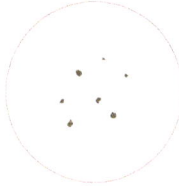

QUINOA

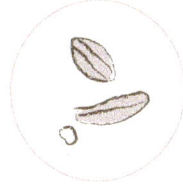

NUTS
(ALMOND, PECAN &
PISTACHIO)

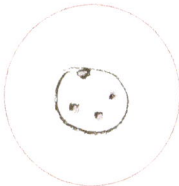

COCONUT

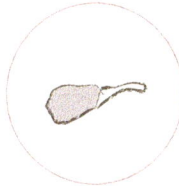

LAMB

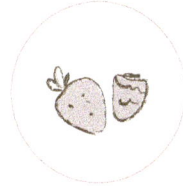

BERRIES
(STRAWBERRY &
RASBERRY)

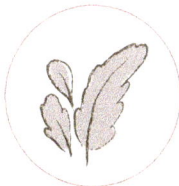

LEAFY GREENS

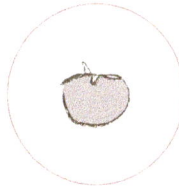

TOMATO

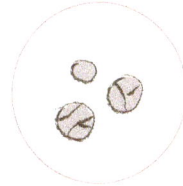

BRUSSEL SPROUTS

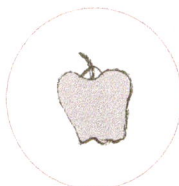

CAPSICUM

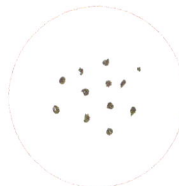

LENTILS

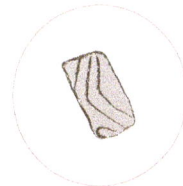

FISH

ovulatory
recipes

# breakfast

Glow & Vitality
Smoothie

Chocolate &
Salted Caramel
Quinoa Porridge

Mediterranean
Frittata

Pink Puddings

Seedy Fruit
Breakfast Bowl

Green Queen
Breakfast Bowl

Creamy Smashed Avo
with Smoked Salmon

# GLOW & VITALITY SMOOTHIE

**Serves:** 1   **Prep:** 5 minutes   **Cook:** N/A

½ cup frozen raspberries
½ cup frozen strawberries
¼ cup frozen pink
  dragonfruit (optional)
1 small fig
1 banana
1 tbsp chia seeds
1 tbsp flaxseeds
1 tbsp pumpkin seeds
1 tbsp almond butter
1 cup coconut milk
1 tsp maca powder
1 heaped tbsp vanilla
  protein powder

Add all the ingredients to a blender and blend until smooth. Serve immediately.

*This recipe also doubles as a snack option.*

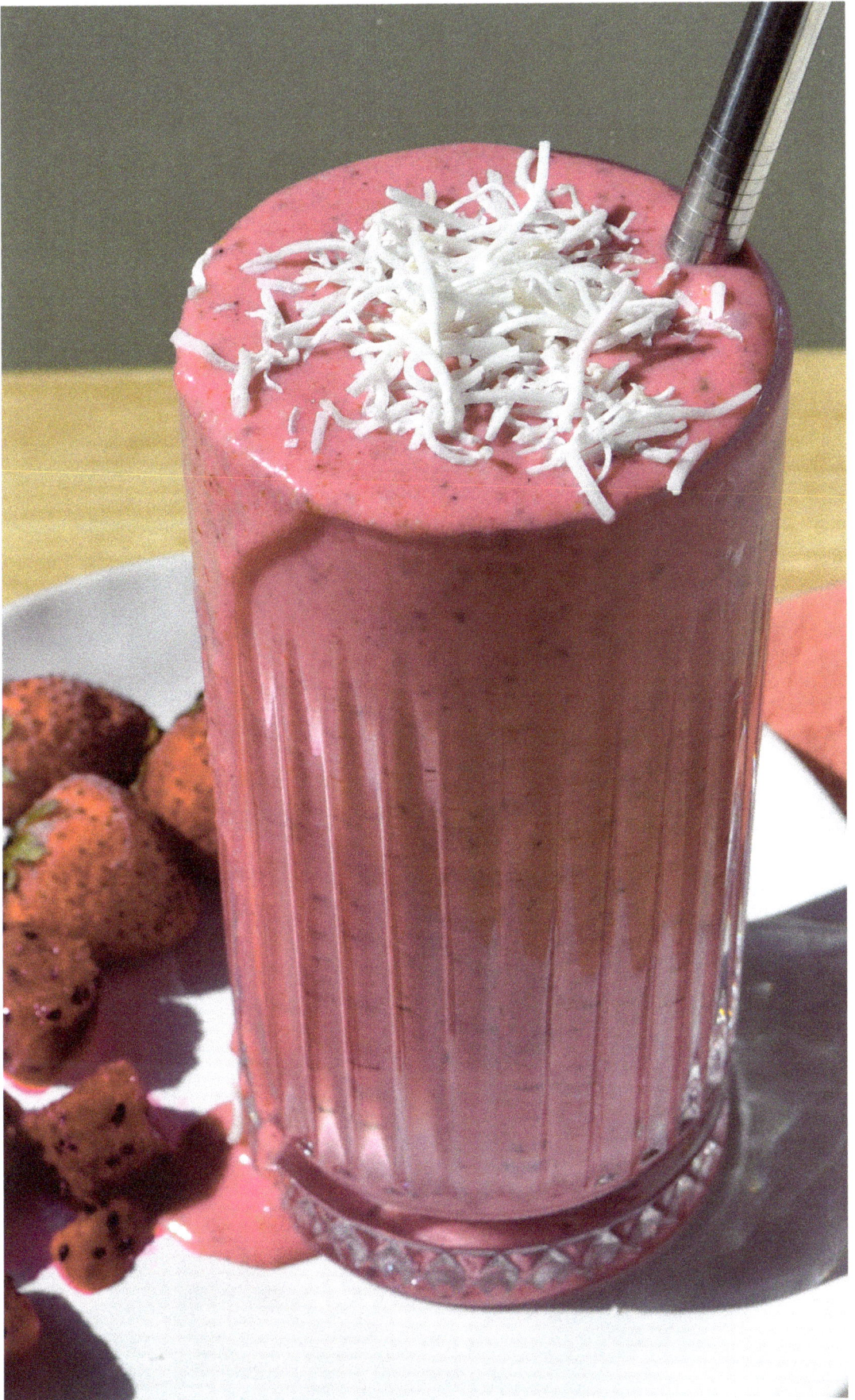

# CHOCOLATE & SALTED CARAMEL QUINOA PORRIDGE

**Serves:** 4    **Prep:** 5 minutes    **Cook:** 15 minutes

½ cup quinoa
¼ cup chia seeds
3 cups water
1 banana, mashed
400ml coconut milk
1 tbsp cacao powder
1 tbsp flaxseed meal

**For the salted caramel sauce:**
1 tbsp tahini
1 tbsp maple syrup
2 tbsp water
Pinch of sea salt

**To serve (per serve):**
½ banana, sliced
1 tbsp almonds, roughly chopped
1 tbsp pecans, roughly chopped
1 tbsp sunflower seeds
1 tbsp pepitas

In a saucepan, add the quinoa, chia seeds and water. Cover with a lid and bring to boil. Remove the lid and reduce to simmer, stirring often until the quinoa is cooked, adding more water if needed.

Add the mashed banana, coconut milk, cacao powder and flaxseed meal. Allow to simmer.

To make the salted caramel sauce, add the tahini, maple syrup, water and salt to a small bowl and whisk until combined.

Serve the quinoa porridge into a bowl and top with fresh banana slices, chopped nuts, seeds, and a drizzle of salted caramel sauce.

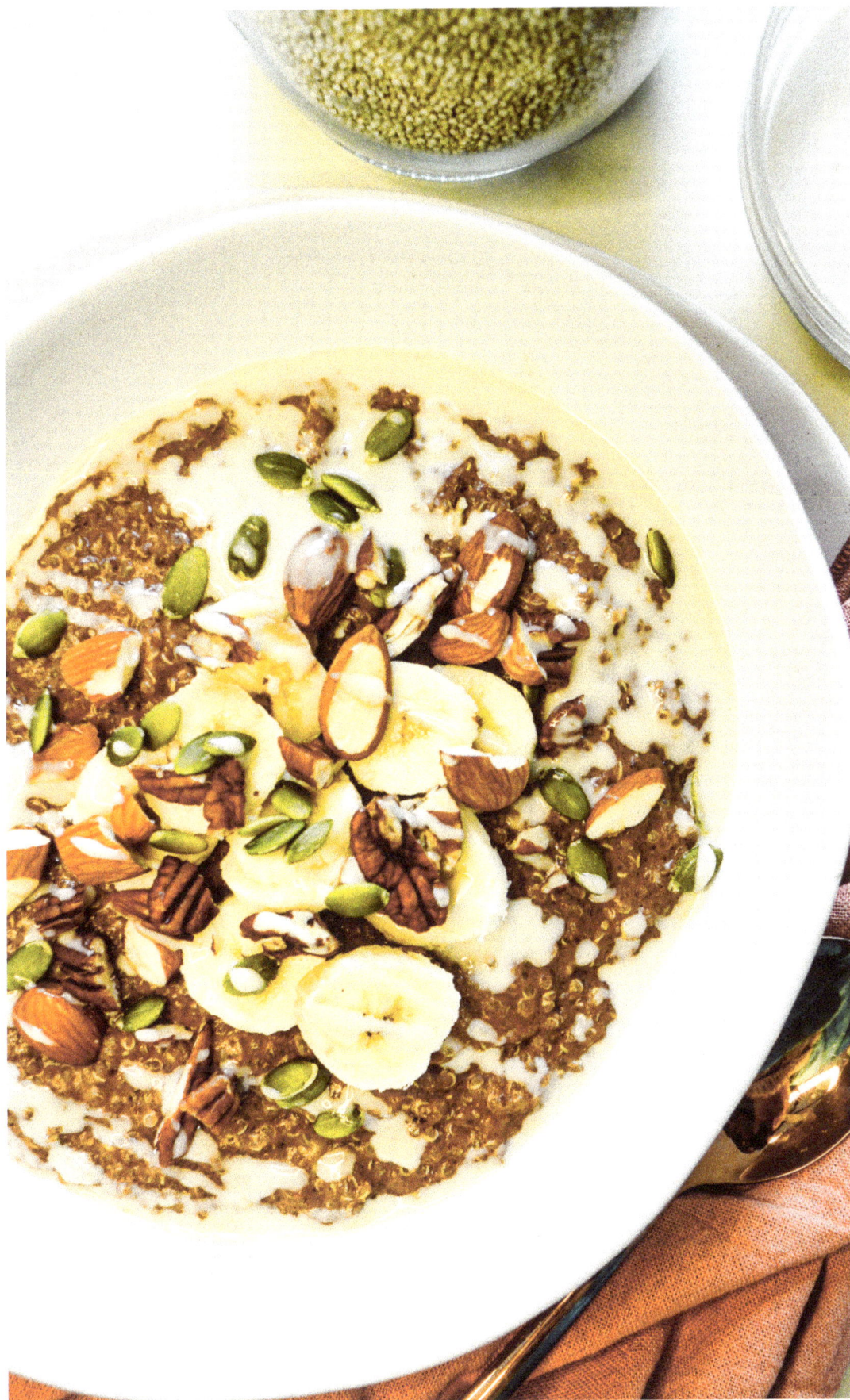

# MEDITERRANEAN FRITTATA

**Serves:** 4    **Prep:** 10 minutes    **Cook:** 40 minutes

2 tsp olive oil
1 cup spinach, chopped
1 capsicum, diced
8 eggs
½ cup milk
1 cup cottage cheese
Salt and pepper, to taste
1 cup cherry tomatoes,
  diced
2 tbsp fresh parsley or basil,
  chopped
½ cup feta cheese,
  crumbled
¼ cup kalamata olives,
  pitted and halved

**Serving suggestions:**
Sourdough bread
Avocado (½ avocado per
  serve)

Preheat the oven to 180°C fan-forced.

In a cast iron pan, heat the olive oil on medium and lightly sauté the spinach and capsicum for 1-2 minutes.

Whisk together the eggs, milk, cottage cheese, salt and pepper in a large bowl until smooth. Stir in tomatoes, herbs of choice, feta and olives.

Pour the egg mixture into the cast iron pan with the sautéed veggies and bake in the oven for 30-35 minutes, or until the centre is set and slightly golden.

Let it cool slightly before slicing into 4 large portions and serving with sourdough bread and avocado.

**NOTE:**
› If you don't have a cast iron pan, sauté the vegetables in a
  normal pan and transfer to a baking dish.

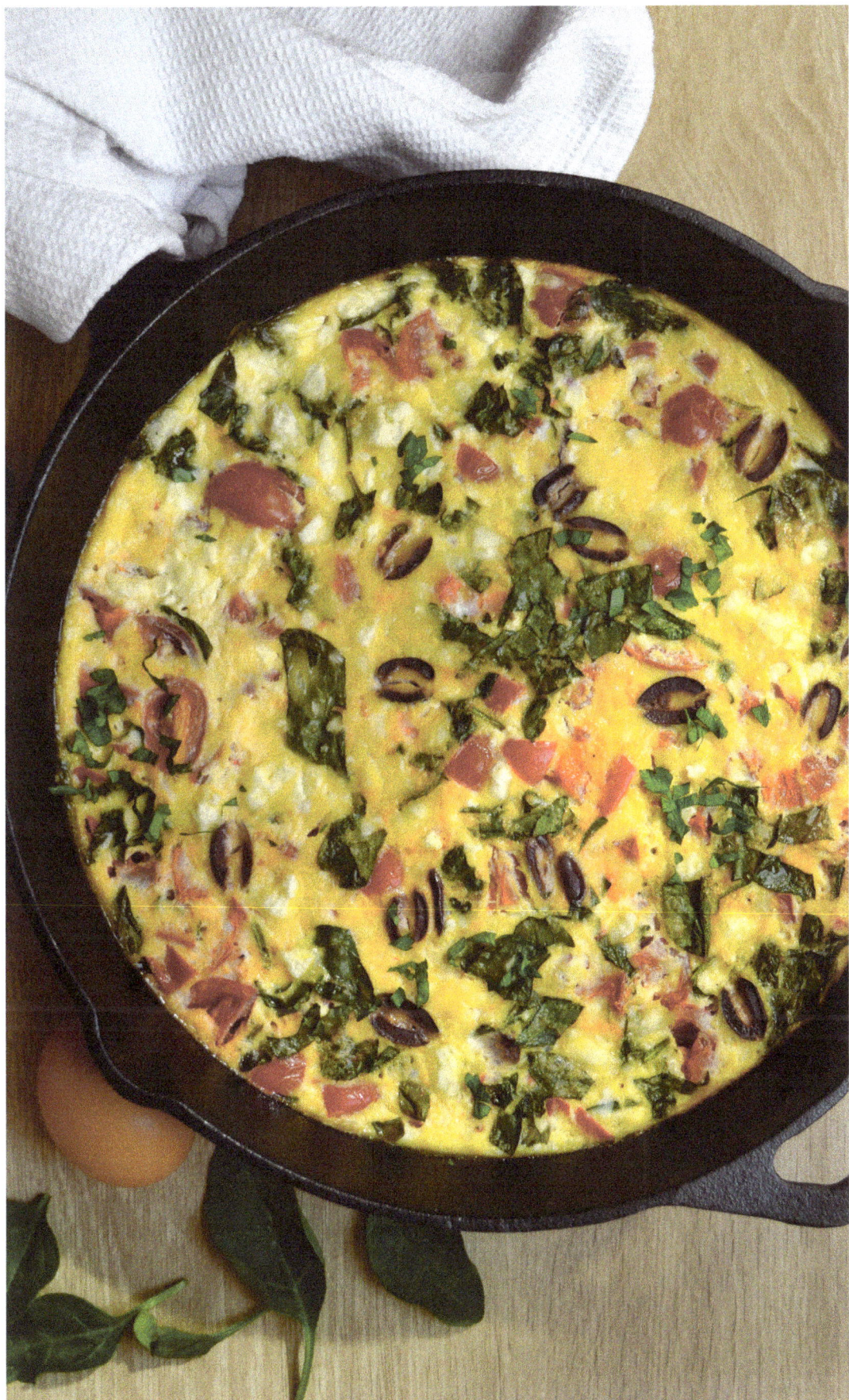

# PINK PUDDINGS

**Serves:** 4    **Prep:** 5 minutes    **Cook:** 4 hours +

½ cup frozen strawberries
¼ cup frozen raspberries
¼ cup frozen pink
  dragonfruit*
¼ cup water
½ cup chia seeds
500g Greek yoghurt*
1 tbsp maple syrup
  (optional)
2 heaped tbsp vanilla
  protein powder

Add the strawberries, raspberries, dragonfruit and water into a food processor and blend until the fruit is pureed.

Add the chia seeds, Greek yoghurt, protein powder, and maple syrup into a bowl and stir to combine. Then add in the fruit puree and mix.

Portion out into separate containers/jars or keep in the large bowl. Cover and refrigerate overnight, or at least 4-5 hours.

Top with extra fruit when served, if desired.

**NOTES:**
› If you want to omit the dragonfruit, substitute them for more raspberries.
› Substitute the Greek yoghurt for canned coconut milk for a dairy-free option.

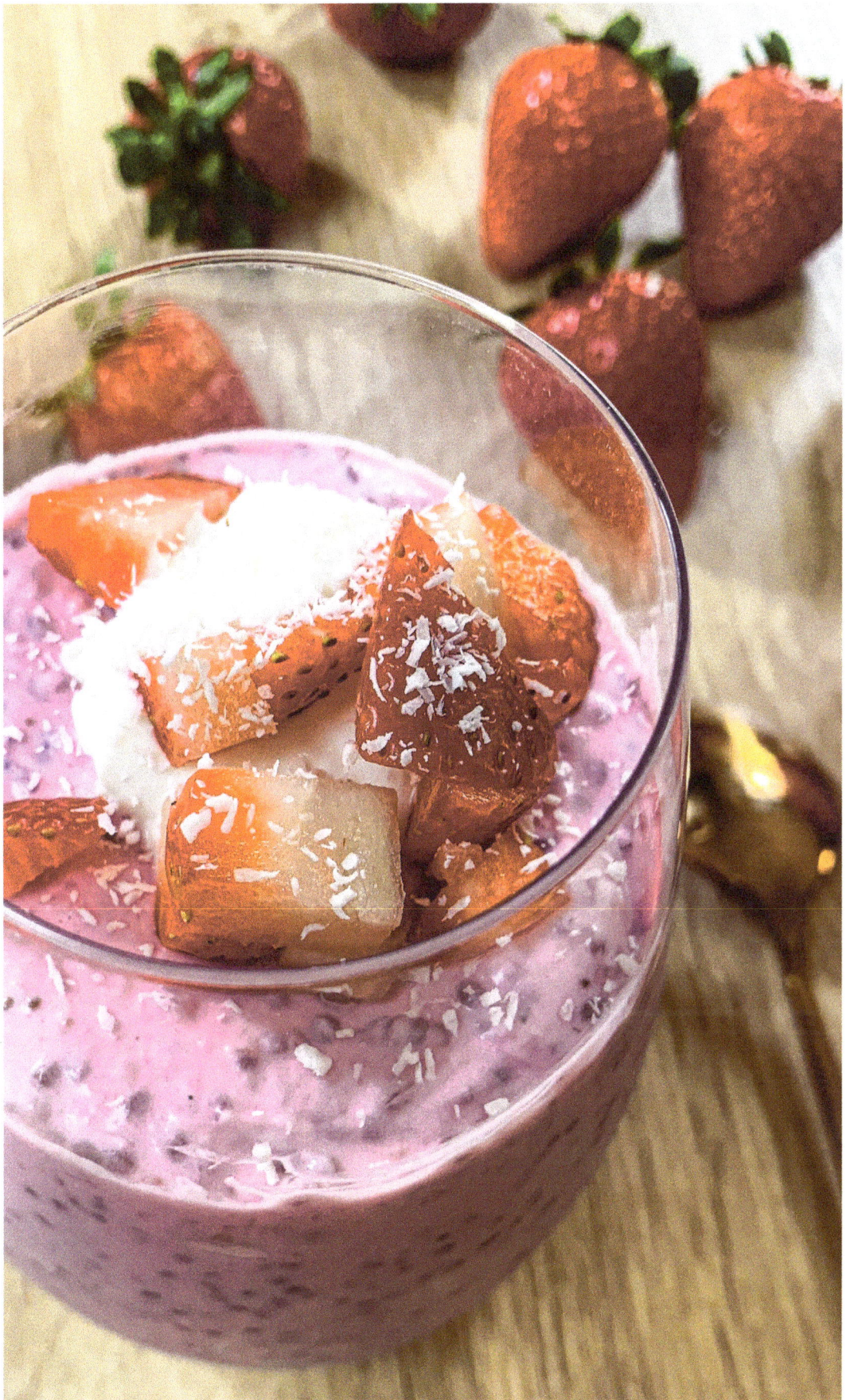

# SEEDY FRUIT BREAKFAST BOWL

**Serves:** 4     **Prep:** 5 minutes     **Cook:** 4 hours +

**For the chia pudding:**
⅓ cup chia seeds
1 cup water
400ml coconut milk

**For the berry compote:**
1 cup frozen berries
½ tsp lemon juice
¼ cup water

**To serve:**
Greek yoghurt
Grain-free granola (see page 255)
Ovulatory phase fruits to choose from: rockmelon, strawberries, blueberries, honeydew melon
Desiccated coconut
Sunflower seeds

Combine the chia seeds, water and coconut milk in a bowl. Cover and refrigerate overnight or for at least 4 hours.

Add the berries, lemon juice and water into a pot on low heat and bring to a simmer. Reduce the heat and cook until berries are soft enough to mash.

To serve, place the yoghurt at the bottom of the bowl, followed by the chia pudding. Then top with fruits, granola, berry compote, desiccated coconut and sunflower seeds.

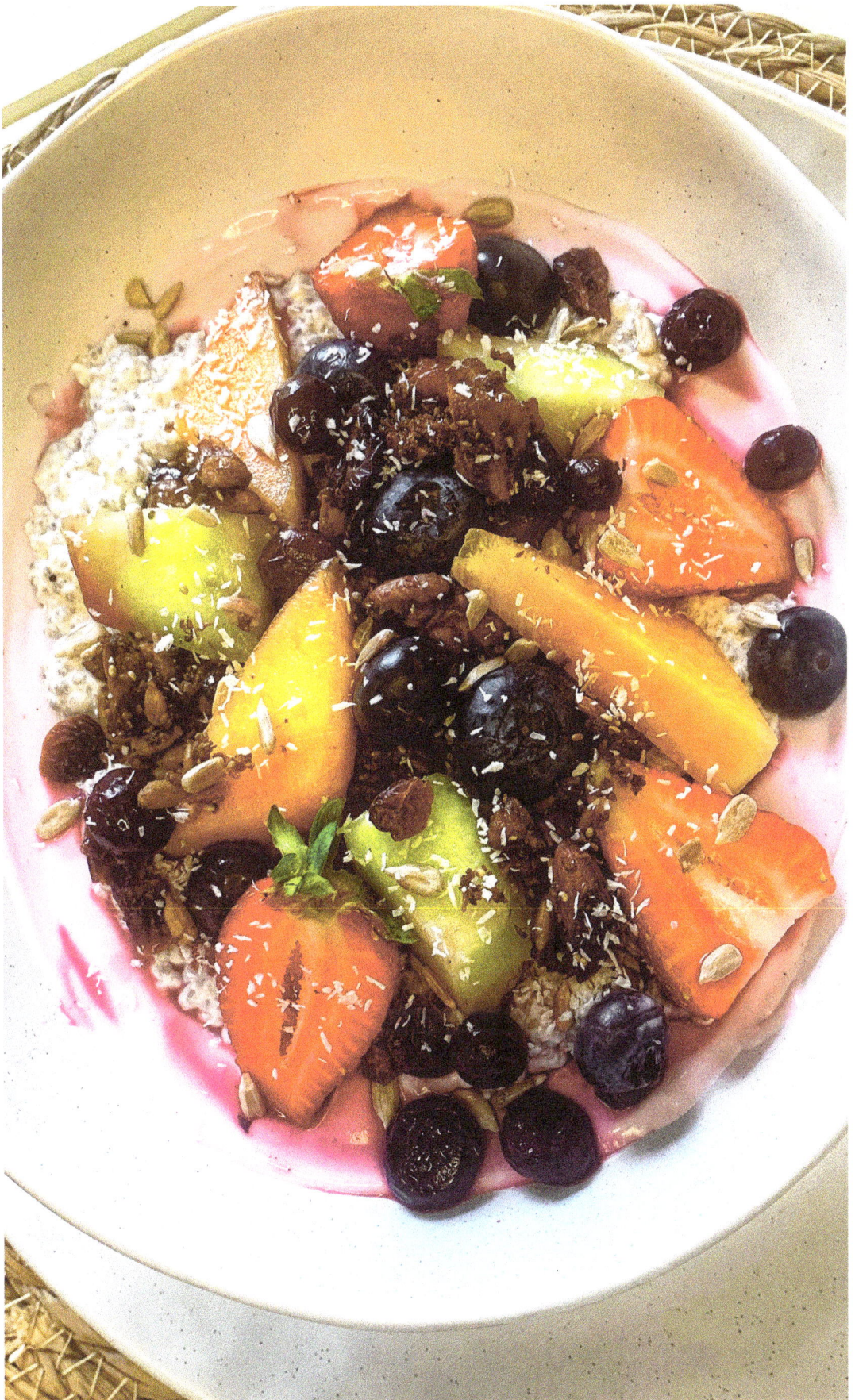

# GREEN QUEEN BREAKFAST BOWL

**Serves:** 4     **Prep:** 10 minutes     **Cook:** 15 minutes

½ cup quinoa
1 ½ cups water
1 tsp olive oil
1 bunch asparagus, halved
   lengthways
1 garlic clove, finely diced
1 lemon, juiced and zested
3 cups kale or spinach,
   roughly chopped
180g halloumi, diced
4 eggs

**For the dressing:**
2 tbsp tahini
1 tbsp maple syrup
1 tbsp olive oil
1 lemon, juiced
2 tbsp water

**To serve:**
¼ cup pomegranate seeds
¼ cup pepita seeds
¼ cup phase friendly nuts
   (brazil, almond, pecan
   or pistachio), roughly
   chopped
½ cup sauerkraut
2 avocadoes, halved

Add the quinoa and water into a pot, cover with a lid and then bring to the boil. Reduce to a simmer and remove the lid, stirring regularly. Cook until the water has evaporated and the quinoa has cooked.

In a pan on low-medium heat, warm the olive oil. Add the asparagus, garlic and lemon juice and zest and cook for 2 minutes until tender. Remove from the pan and set aside. Add the kale/spinach to the pan and cook for 2–3 minutes until wilted. Remove and set aside.

In the same pan, add the halloumi and cook for 3–4 minutes until lightly golden. Set aside.

Bring a pot of water to a boil, add the eggs and boil for 7 minutes (for a soft boiled egg). Remove and add to a bowl of cold water before peeling and setting aside.

Add the tahini, maple syrup, olive oil, lemon juice and water in a jar and stir until smooth and creamy. Adjust the water according to your consistency preference.

Build your breakfast bowl by dividing the quinoa, kale, asparagus, halloumi and eggs equally across four bowls. Top with pomegranate seeds, pepita seeds, chosen nuts, sauerkraut and avocado. Drizzle the dressing over the top and serve.

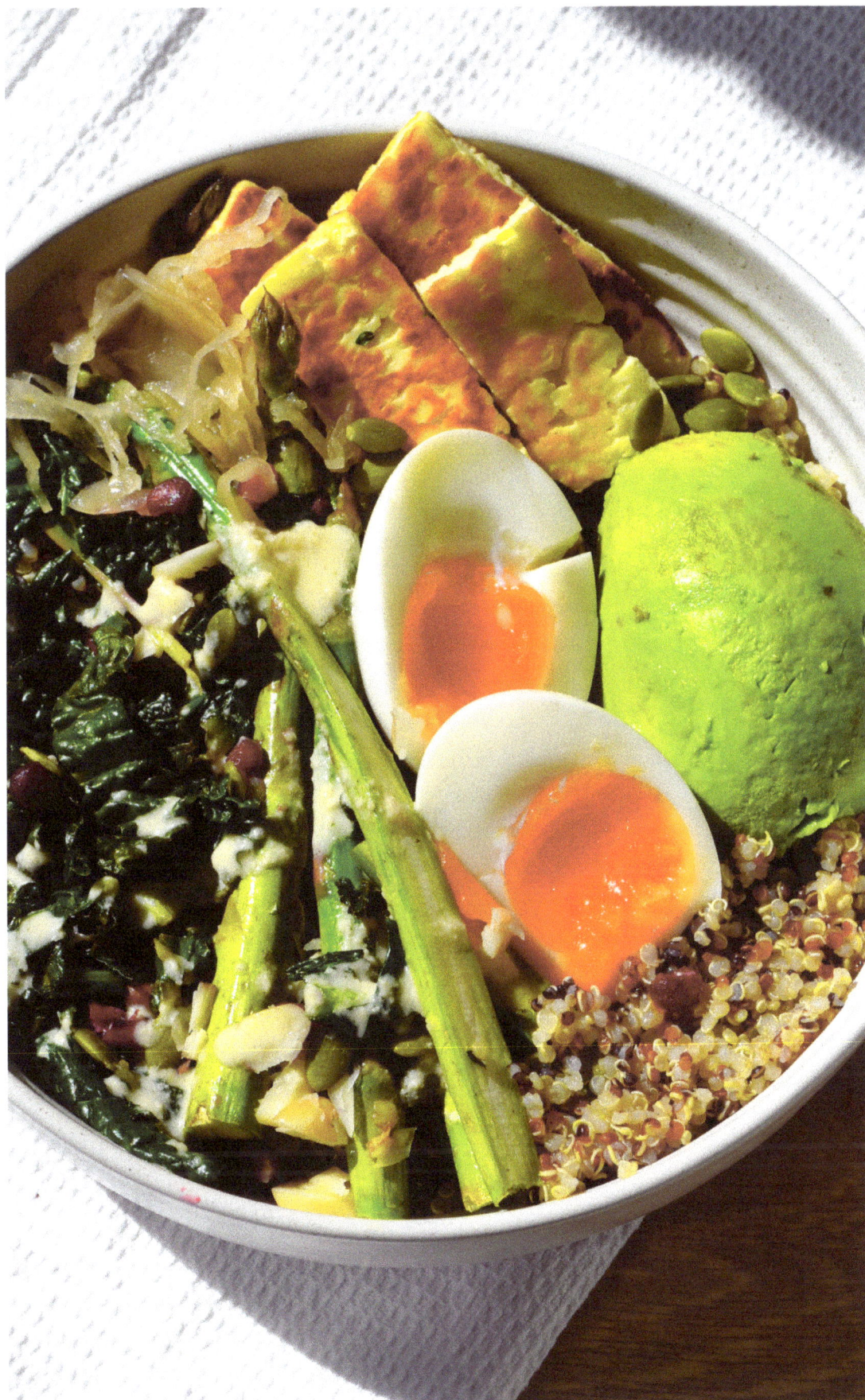

# CREAMY SMASHED AVO
## WITH SMOKED SALMON

**Serves:** 1　　**Prep:** 5 minutes　　**Cook:** N/A

½ avocado
½ cup cottage cheese
Salt and pepper
2 tbsp fresh dill, chopped
½ lemon, juiced
2 pieces of toasted
　sourdough, or bread of
　choice
50g smoked salmon

**Optional toppings:**
Red onion
Capers
Fresh dill
Poached eggs

In a bowl, add the avocado and mash. Then add the cottage cheese, salt and pepper, dill and lemon juice.

Assemble by placing the slices of toast onto the plate and spreading the avocado and cottage cheese mix on top. Top with smoked salmon and garnish with extra dill, red onion and capers, if desired.

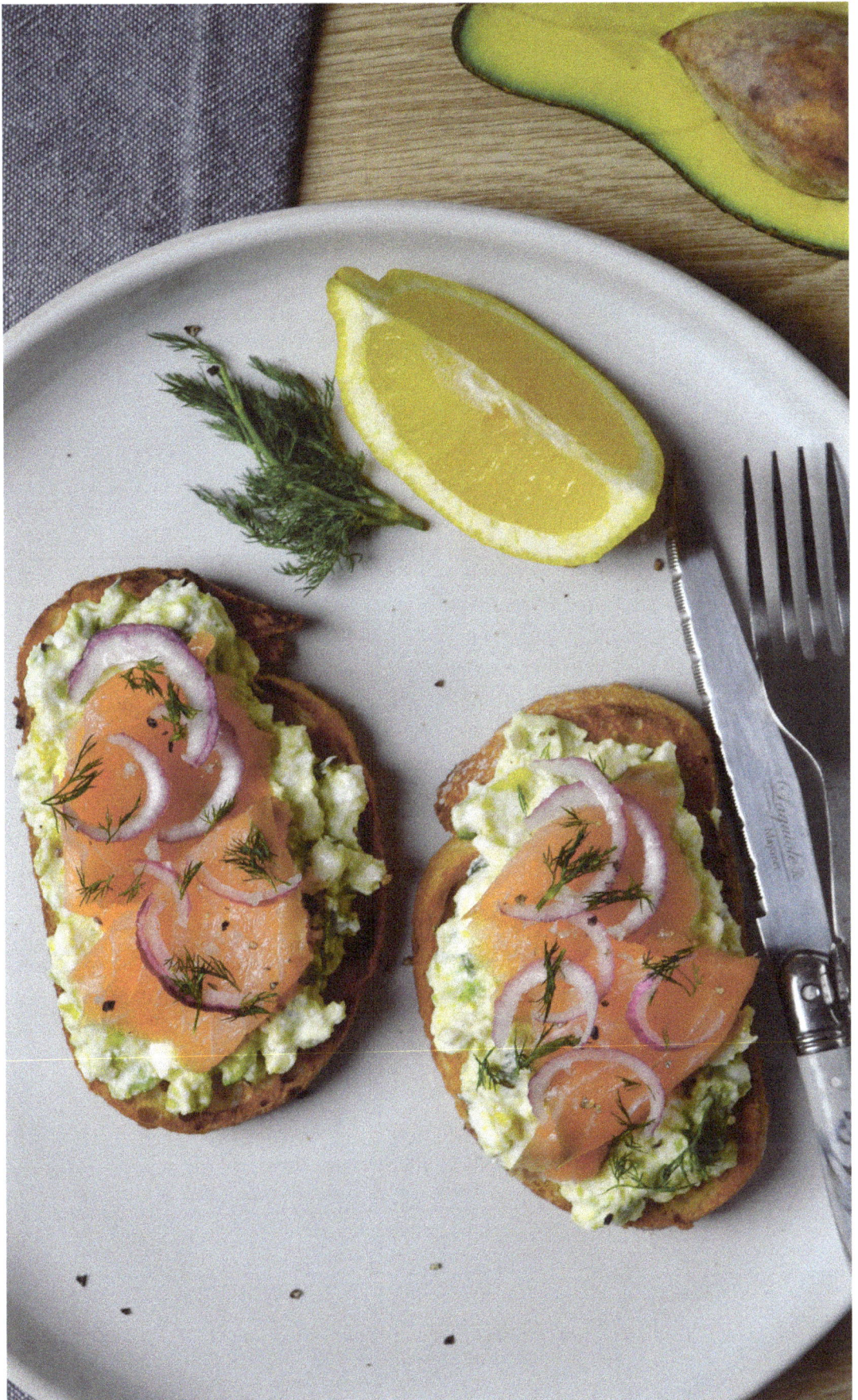

# mains

Tuna &
Lentil Salad

Veggie &
Halloumi Stacks

Salmon
all'Arrabbiata

Lamb Steaks
with Baba
Ganoush & Greens

Lamb Souvlaki
Lettuce Cups

Fresh Tuna Steaks
with Asian Greens

Lamb Salad

Nicoise Nourish Bowl

Salmon &
Couscous Salad

Tandoori
Salmon Salad

# TUNA & LENTIL SALAD

**Serves:** 4    **Prep:** 10 minutes    **Cook:** N/A

3 cups spinach, chopped
3-4 tomatoes, diced
2 red capsicums, diced
2 cucumbers, halved and
  sliced
⅓ cup kalamata olives,
  roughly chopped
1 tbsp capers (optional)
400g brown lentils, drained
  and rinsed
4 cans tuna in springwater,
  drained (1 can per serve)

**For the dressing:**
1 lemon, juiced
1 tbsp apple cider vinegar
¼ cup olive oil
1 tbsp Dijon mustard

Combine all the vegetables in a bowl, then add the lentils and tuna when serving.

For the dressing, combine the lemon juice, apple cider vinegar, olive oil and Dijon mustard in a jar/bowl and mix well.

When ready to serve, add the dressing to the salad and toss to combine.

**TIP:**
› If serving later or meal prepping, add the tuna in at the same time as the dressing to avoid the vegetables going soggy.

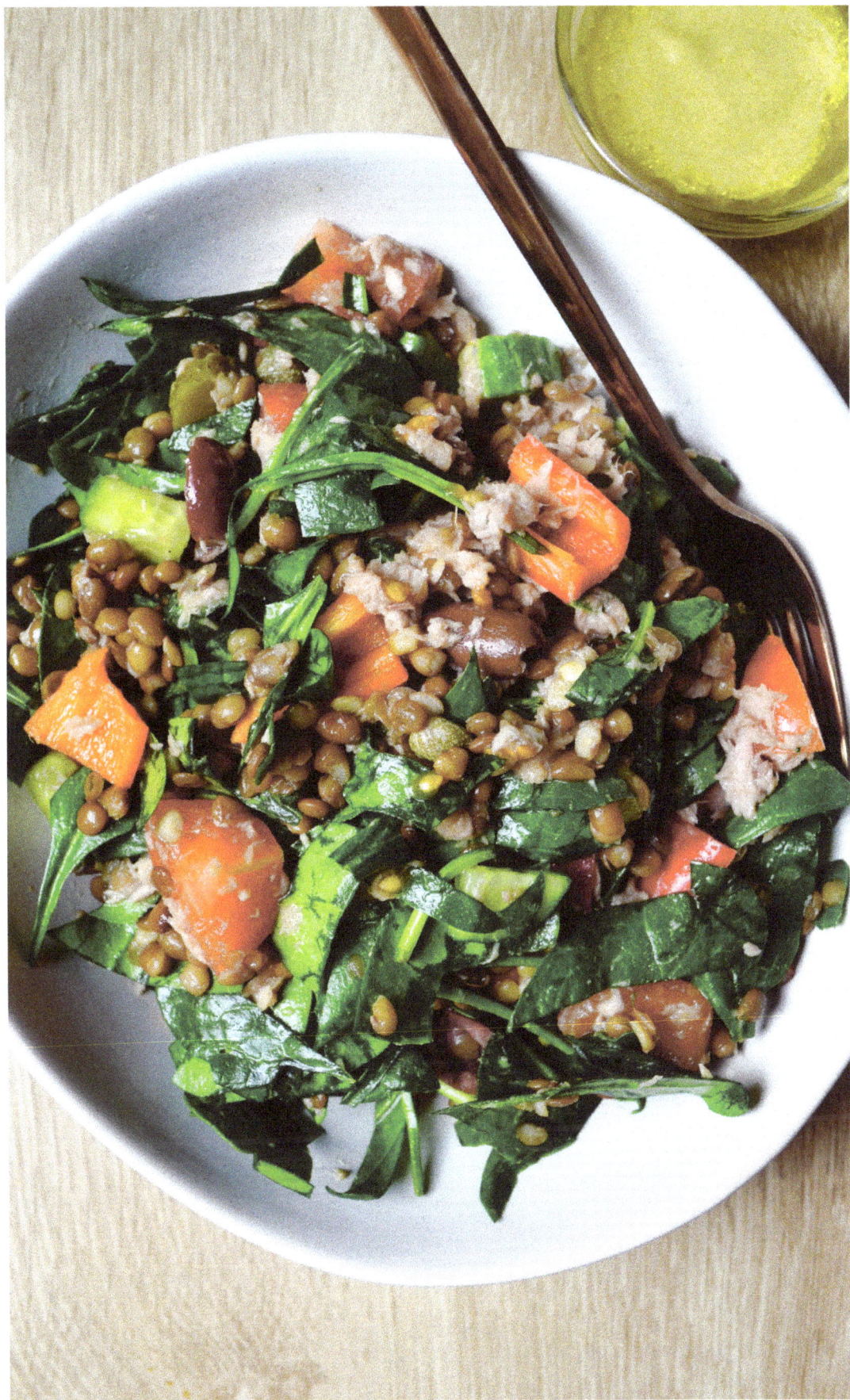

# VEGGIE & HALLOUMI STACKS

**Serves:** 4    **Prep:** 15 minutes    **Cook:** 35 minutes

1 large eggplant, sliced
1 sweet potato, peeled and
  sliced lengthways
1 zucchini, halved and sliced
  lengthways
Olive oil
Salt and pepper
3-4 white mushrooms,
  sliced
1 red onion, sliced
2 cups passata
1 cup spinach
1 block halloumi, sliced
1 cup grated cheese

Preheat the oven to 180°C fan-forced and line two
baking trays.

Slice the eggplant lengthways, creating "steak-like" pieces.
Sprinkle salt on both sides of the eggplant and leave to rest
on a paper towel to absorb excess water.

Slice and prepare the remaining vegetables and halloumi.

Place the sweet potato and zucchini on the baking trays,
drizzle with olive oil and season with salt and pepper. Bake in
the oven for about 30 minutes until soft.

Heat a fry pan or grill on medium with a little olive oil and
cook the eggplant, mushrooms and onions in batches.

Once all are cooked, assemble the stacks on the baking trays.
Begin with the eggplant, then add a tablespoon of passata
and spread it over the top of the eggplant. Add the spinach,
halloumi, sweet potato, zucchini, mushrooms and onions.
Add another tablespoon of passata and top with some
grated cheese. Repeat the process until all the eggplant
steaks have been used.

Return the trays to the oven and bake the stacks for
5 minutes or until the cheese has melted.

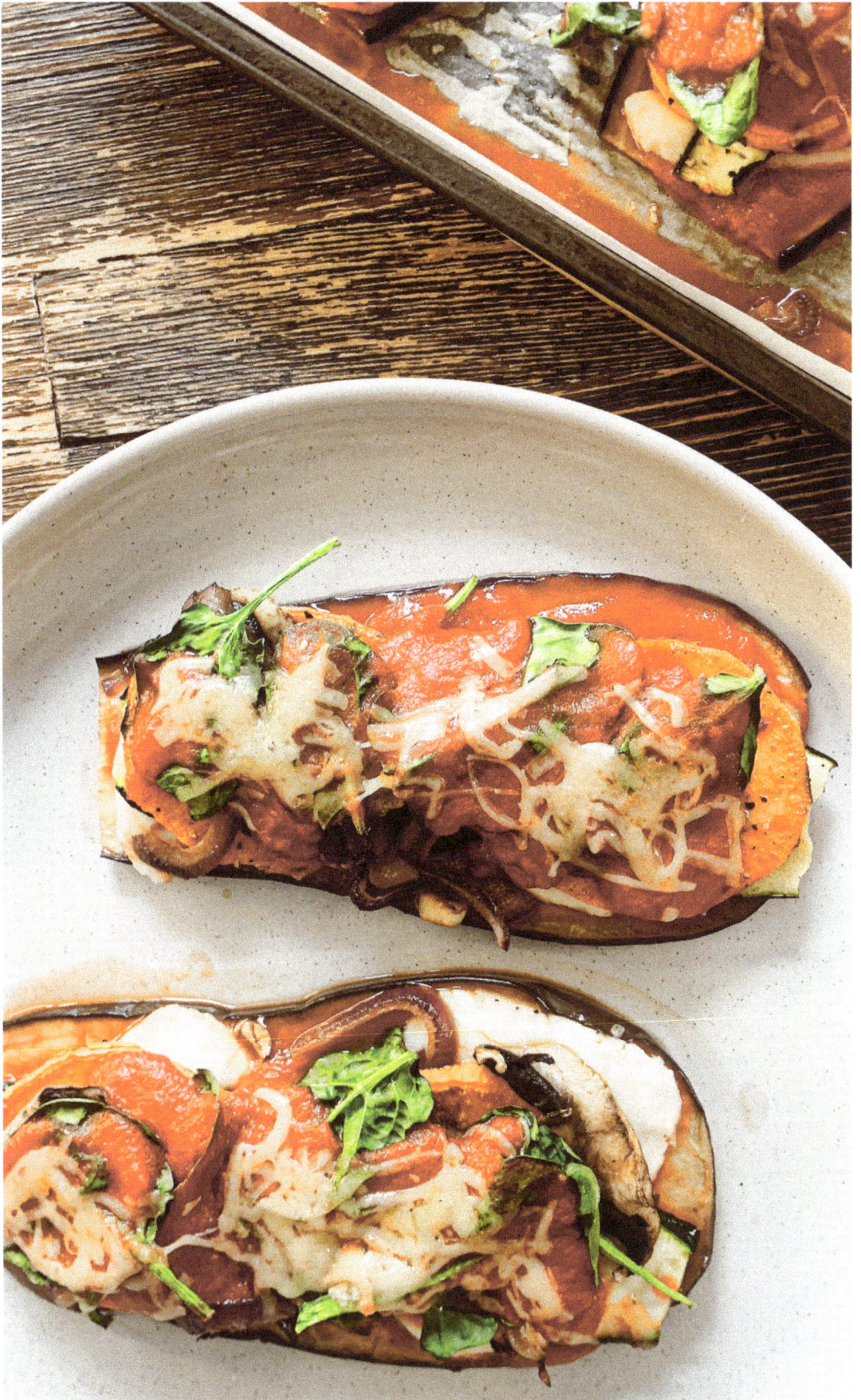

# SALMON ALL'ARRABBIATA

**Serves:** 4    **Prep:** 10 minutes    **Cook:** 30 minutes

1 tsp olive oil
1 onion, finely chopped
2 cloves garlic, chopped
½ red chilli, finely chopped
2 tbsp tomato paste
1 tbsp dried oregano
½ tsp dried ground sage
700ml passata
½ cup water
1 tbsp red wine vinegar
1 tbsp balsamic vinegar
¼ cup kalamata olives,
  sliced
2 tsp capers
2 cups spinach, chopped
4 salmon fillets, skin off

**For the greens:**
1 tsp olive oil
1 garlic clove, sliced
2 asparagus bunches, sliced
  in half lengthways
1 lemon, juiced

**To serve:**
Risoni pasta, cooked (1 cup
  per serve)

In a pan on medium heat, add the olive oil, onion and garlic and cook until the onion is translucent. Then mix in the chilli, tomato paste, oregano and ground sage and stir.

Add the passata, water, vinegars, olives and capers.

Simmer for 10 minutes. Add the spinach. Then add the salmon fillets. Cover for about 10-15 minutes or until the salmon has cooked through to your liking.

In another heated pan with olive oil, add the sliced garlic and sauté for 1 minute. Then add the asparagus and lemon juice, cooking for 3-5 minutes until the asparagus has softened slightly.

Serve the salmon and sauce with the asparagus and risoni pasta.

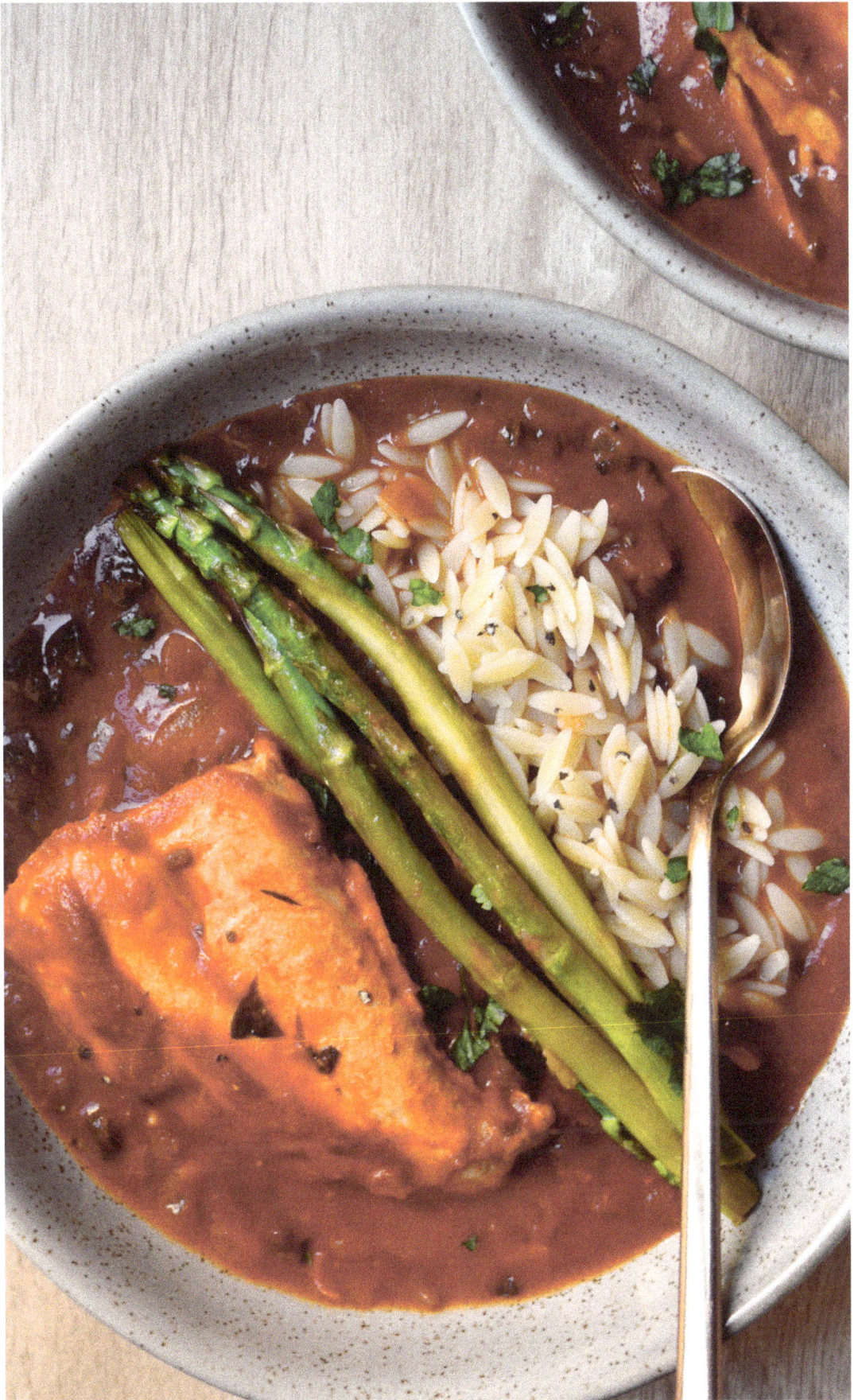

# LAMB STEAKS
## WITH BABA GANOUSH & GREENS

**Serves:** 2     **Prep:** 5 minutes     **Cook:** 40 minutes

1 lamb backstrap (approx. 200g), seasoned as desired

**For the baba ganoush:**
2 eggplants, sliced lengthways
2 tbsp tahini
1 tbsp olive oil
1 ½ tbsp smoked paprika (adjusted to taste)
1 garlic clove
½ cup water
1 lemon, juiced

**For the greens:**
½ tbsp olive oil
1 bunch asparagus
1 ½ cups brussel sprouts, halved
1 garlic clove, finely chopped
1 lemon, zested and juiced
¼ cup parsley, chopped
¼ cup pistachios, roughly chopped

Preheat the oven to 200°C fan-forced.

On a lined baking tray, place the eggplants flesh side up and roast for 30 minutes. Remove and allow to cool before peeling off the skins.

In a food processor, add the eggplant flesh, tahini, olive oil, smoked paprika, garlic, water and lemon. Blend until smooth. Set aside.

To make the greens, heat an oven-safe frypan on medium with a drizzle of olive oil. Add the asparagus and brussel sprouts and sauté for 3 minutes. Add the garlic and lemon juice and sauté for another 3 minutes or until tender. Transfer the pan to the oven and bake for 8-10 minutes. Serve with lemon zest, parsley and pistachios.

Cook the lamb steaks in a frypan on medium heat with olive oil according to your desired tenderness.

Serve steaks on a bed of warm baba ganoush and serve with the greens.

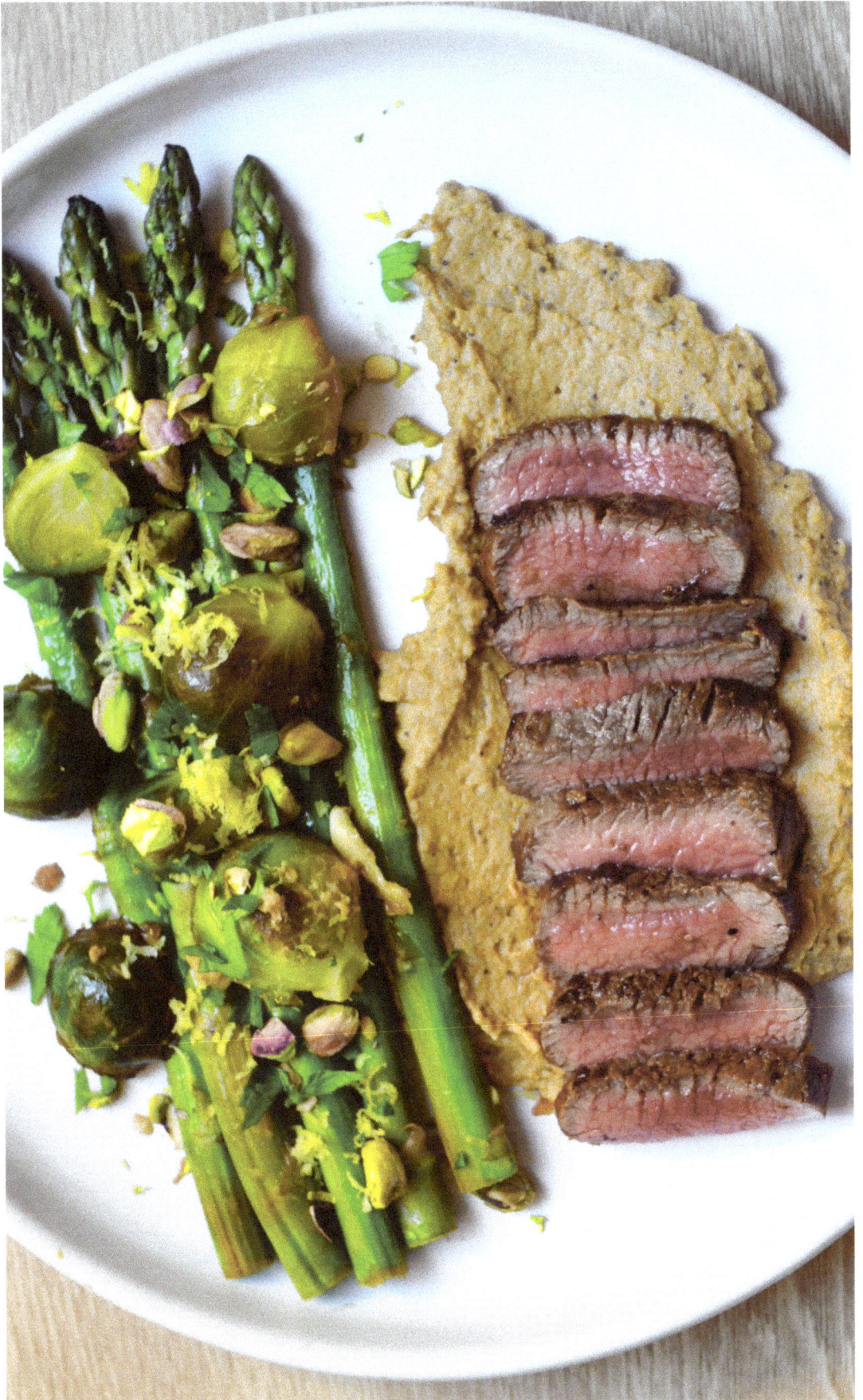

# LAMB SOUVLAKI LETTUCE CUPS

**Serves:** 2    **Prep:** 10 minutes    **Cook:** 5 minutes

300g lamb strips
2 tbsp oregano
1 tbsp olive oil
½ lemon, juiced
1 garlic clove, crushed
Pinch of salt and pepper
1 lettuce head, leaves
  separated
2 tomatoes, diced
1 cucumber, diced
Red onion, sliced

**For the tzatziki dip:**
1 cup Greek yoghurt
½ cucumber, grated (excess
  water squeezed out)
½ lemon, juiced

**Serving suggestion:**
2 wholemeal pita pockets,
  toasted
Feta

Add the lamb, oregano, olive oil, lemon juice, garlic, salt and pepper into a bowl and stir to combine. Stand aside, allowing it to marinate.

To make the dip, combine the yoghurt, grated cucumber and lemon juice in a small bowl. Mix to combine.

In a frypan on medium heat, cook the lamb in batches (to avoid stewing) for 1-2 minutes. Remove from heat and allow them to rest.

Serve by placing the lamb strips in the lettuce cups, along with the tomato, cucumber, red onion and dip.

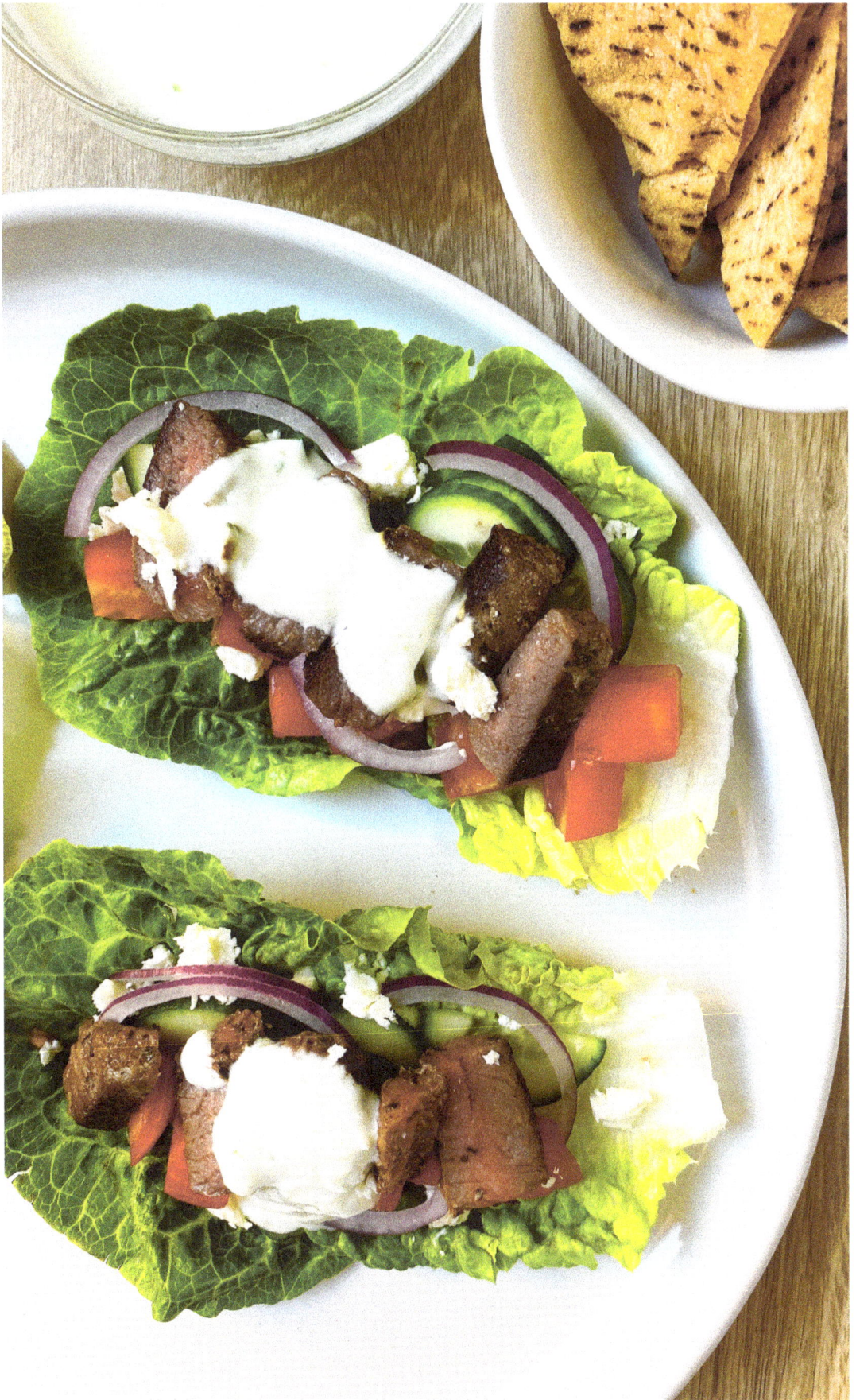

# FRESH TUNA STEAKS
## WITH ASIAN GREENS

**Serves:** 2      **Prep:** 10 minutes      **Cook:** 10 minutes

2 tbsp black sesame seeds
2 tbsp white sesame seeds
1 lime, zested (use juice for
   the greens)
2 tuna steaks
1 tsp soy sauce/tamari

**For the Asian greens:**
1 tsp olive oil
1 broccolini bunch, chopped
1 bok choy bunch, chopped
1 garlic clove, grated
1 tbsp ginger, grated
1 lime, juiced

**To serve:**
Rice, cooked (optional)
1 cucumber, sliced

Combine the sesame seeds and lime zest in a bowl and set aside.

Lightly brush the tuna steaks with soy sauce/tamari, then coat the steaks in the sesame and lime mixture.

In a pan on medium heat, add olive oil and sauté the broccolini, bok choy, garlic and ginger until the bok choy has slightly wilted. Add the lime juice. Remove from the pan and set aside.

In the same pan, add the tuna steaks. Sear each side for 45-60 seconds, followed by searing around the edges. Depending on the thickness of the steak, it may need a little longer.

Remove from the pan to a chopping board and slice on a slight angle.

Serve on a bed of rice (if desired) with some sliced cucumber. Garnish with additional sesame seeds if desired.

**NOTE:**
› Adjust cooking times based on the thickness of the tuna steaks
  and your preferred level of doneness.

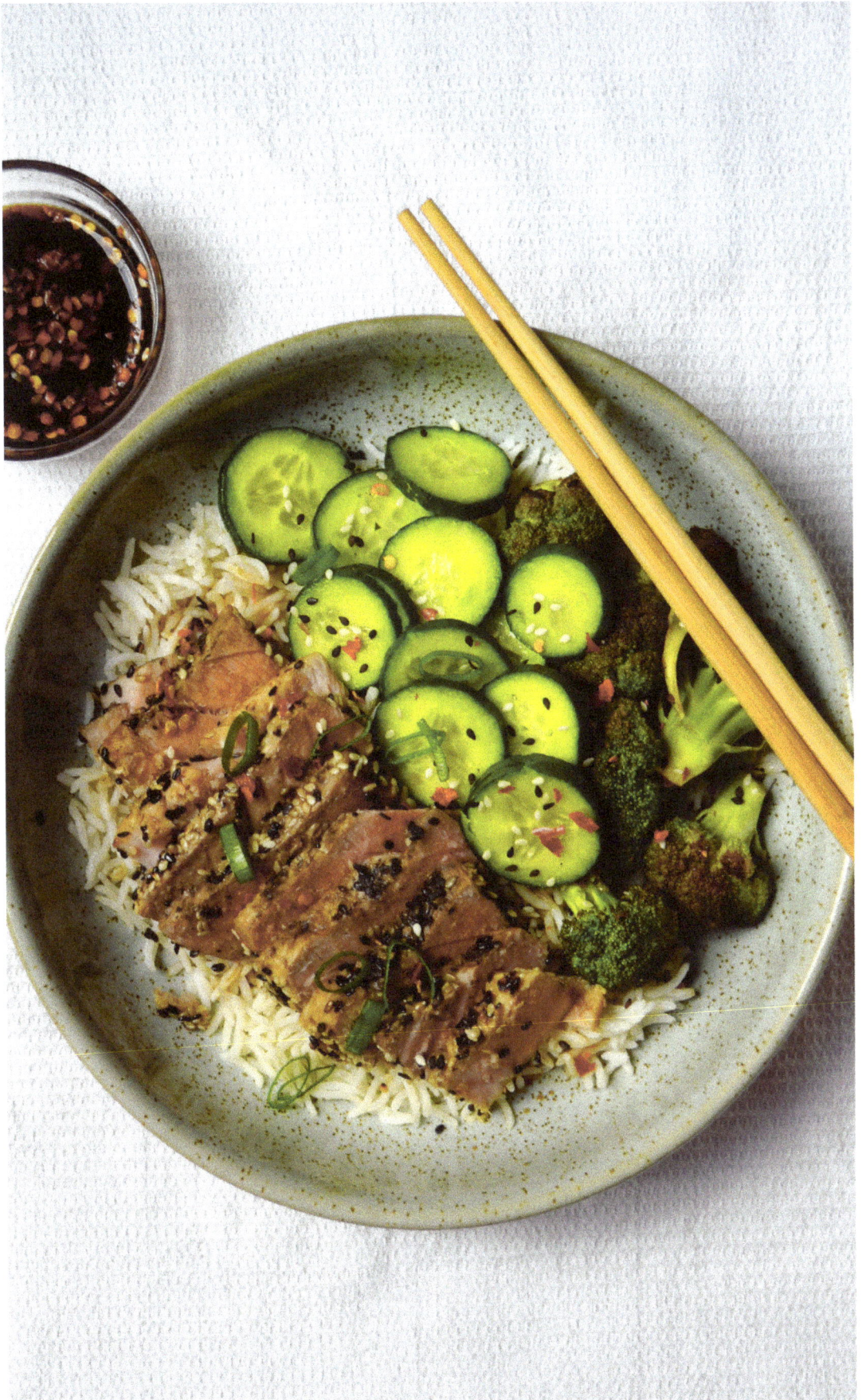

# LAMB SALAD

**Serves:** 2     **Prep:** 10 minutes     **Cook:** 25 minutes

1 sweet potato, peeled and
   diced
Olive oil
Salt and pepper
120g spinach and rocket
   mix
1 cup cherry tomatoes,
   halved
1 cucumber, sliced
1 red capsicum, diced
¼ cup kalamata olives,
   sliced
¼ cup pomegranate seeds
¼ cup feta/goat cheese
1 piece of lamb backstrap

For the yoghurt dressing:
½ cup Greek yoghurt
1 tsp honey
¼ tsp cumin

Preheat the oven to 200°C fan-forced.

Line a baking tray and add the sweet potato. Drizzle with olive oil and season with salt and pepper. Bake in the oven for 20 minutes.

Meanwhile, prepare the salad mix in a large bowl by adding the spinach, rocket, tomatoes, cucumber, capsicum, olives, pomegranate seeds and feta.

In a small bowl, make the dressing by combining the yoghurt, honey and cumin. Set aside.

Prepare the lamb by drizzling it with olive oil and seasoning with salt and pepper on both sides.

In the last 10 minutes of the sweet potato baking, heat a frypan on medium heat. Add the lamb and cook for 4 minutes on each side for a medium-rare tenderness (or to your preferred tenderness). Remove from heat and rest on a plate for 5 minutes. Slice into strips and add to the salad mix.

Remove the sweet potato from the oven and add to the salad mix. Stir through the yoghurt dressing and serve.

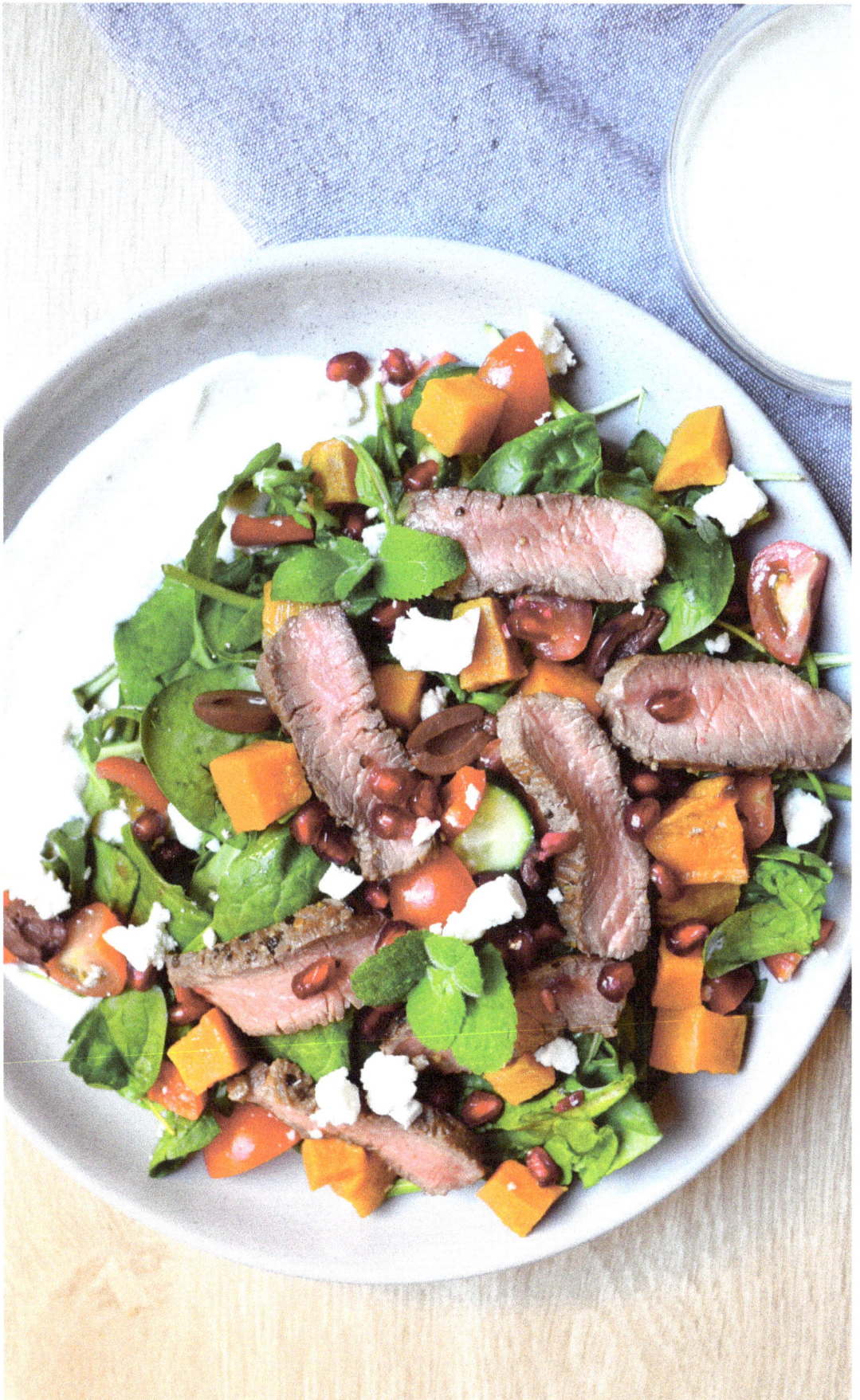

# NICOISE NOURISH BOWL

**Serves:** 4    **Prep:** 10 minutes    **Cook:** 15 minutes

4 eggs
2 white potatoes, thickly
  diced
800g canned lentils,
  drained and rinsed
4 cans tuna in springwater,
  drained
2 cups cherry tomatoes
2 cucumbers, sliced
1 bunch asparagus spears,
  quartered
½ cup kalamata olives
¼ cup capers

**For the dressing:**
⅓ cup olive oil
1 tbsp Dijon mustard
¼ cup red wine vinegar
Salt and pepper to season

Bring a pot of water to boil and boil the eggs to your liking (6 minutes for a soft-boiled egg, 7 minutes for a semi-soft-boiled egg or 10–12 for hard). Place the boiled eggs in a bowl of iced water and peel off the shell.

While the eggs are boiling, add a steaming basket on top and add the diced potatoes. Cover the basket with a lid and steam until tender and a knife easily pierces through. Remove from steaming basket and season with pepper, if desired.

Meanwhile, add the olive oil, mustard, vinegar and salt and pepper to a jar. Cover with a lid and shake until combined.

Build the bowl by adding the lentils, then top with the tuna, tomatoes, cucumber, potatoes, asparagus, olives and capers. Drizzle with dressing when ready to eat.

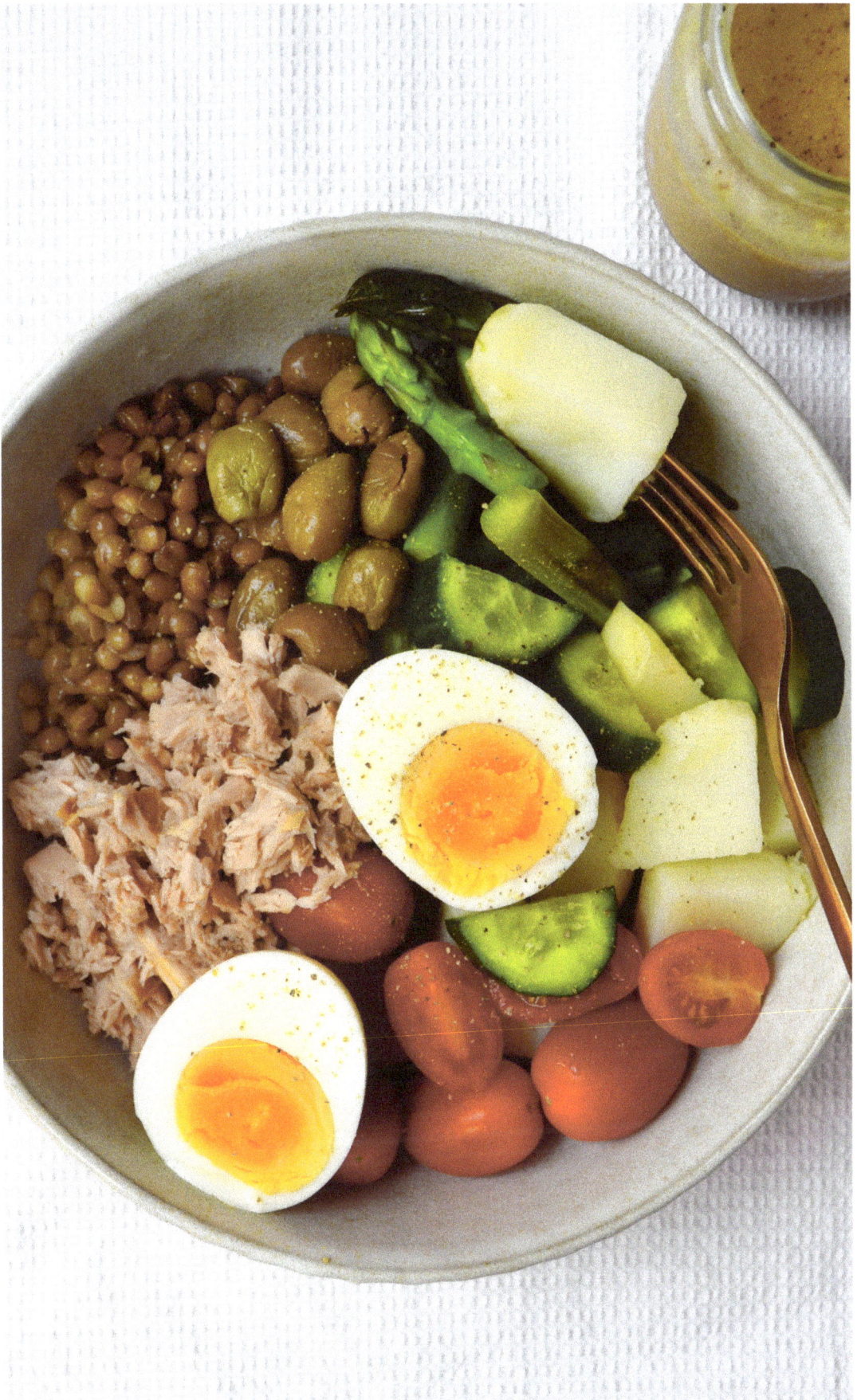

# SALMON & COUSCOUS SALAD

**Serves:** 4     **Prep:** 10 minutes     **Cook:** 20 minutes

2 salmon fillets
200g pearl couscous,
  cooked
3 cups spinach, chopped
1 avocado, diced
2 cucumbers, diced
1 red onion, finely diced
400g canned cannellini
  beans, drained and rinsed
1 cup parsley, chopped
1 cup dill, chopped

**For the honey mustard dressing:**
2 tsp Dijon mustard
1 tbsp olive oil
1 tsp apple cider vinegar
1 tbsp water
1 tbsp honey
A pinch of pepper

Pre-heat the oven to 180°C fan-forced and line a baking tray. Place the salmon on the tray and bake in the oven for 15-20 minutes or until cooked to your liking.

Remove from oven and flake apart using a fork.

Cook the pearl couscous according to packet instructions.

In a small jar, combine the mustard, olive oil, vinegar, water, honey and pepper to make the dressing. Shake to combine well.

In a large bowl, add the spinach, avocado, cucumber, onion, cannellini beans, parsley and dill. Add the couscous and salmon once cooked.

When ready to serve, add the dressing and stir to combine.

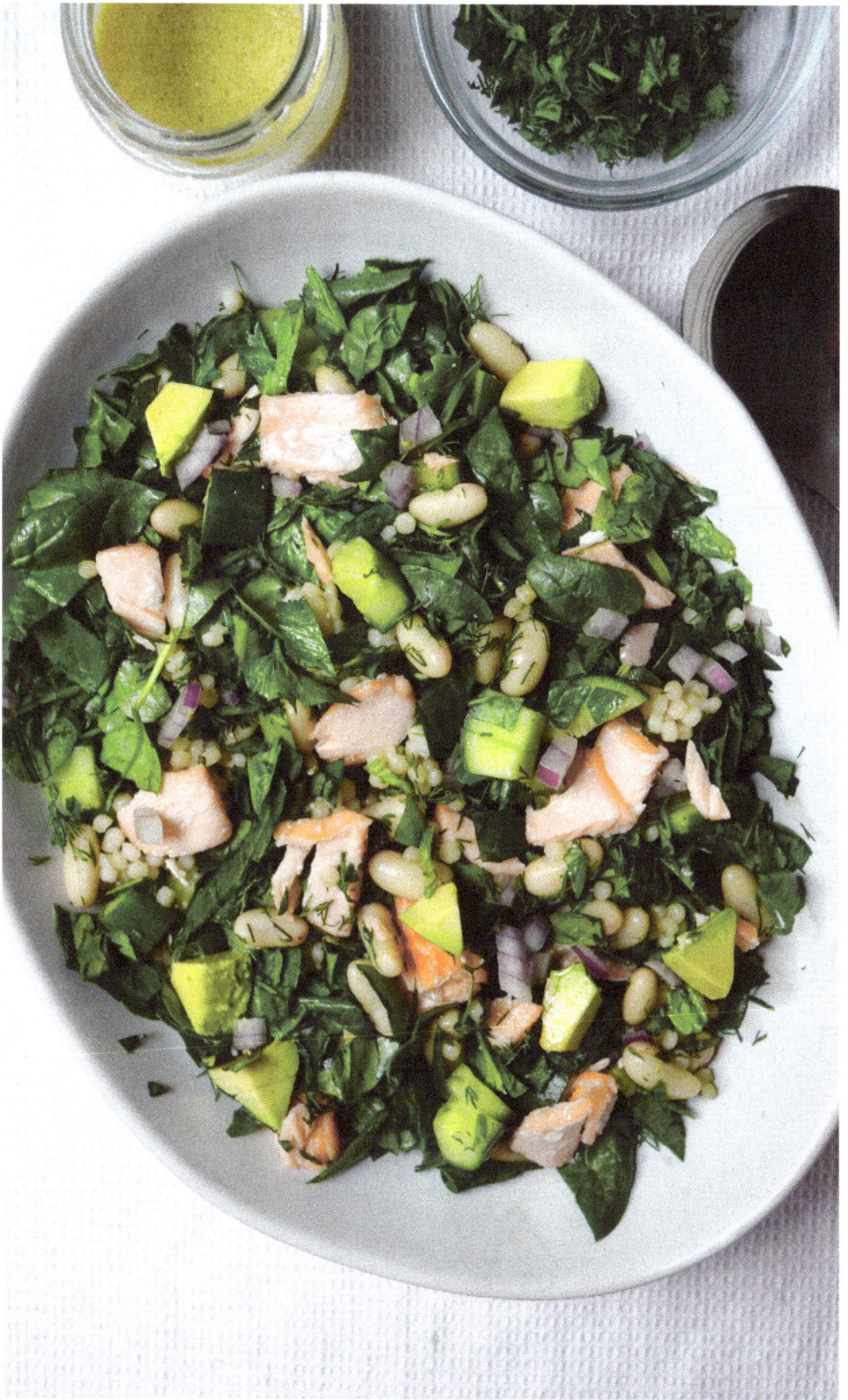

# TANDOORI SALMON SALAD

**Serves:** 4     **Prep:** 10 minutes     **Cook:** 20 minutes

**For the salmon:**
2 tbsp Greek yoghurt
1 tbsp garam masala
1 tsp turmeric
1 tsp cumin
1 tbsp ground paprika
1 tbsp tomato paste
4 salmon fillets, skin off

**For the salad:**
2 heads baby cos lettuce,
  roughly chopped
250g cherry tomatoes,
  quartered
1 cucumber, sliced
1 red onion, finely sliced*

**For the dressing:**
1 cup Greek yoghurt
½ cucumber, grated
1 lemon, juiced

Preheat the oven to 180°C fan-forced. Line a baking tray.

To make the salmon marinade, combine the Greek yoghurt, garam masala, turmeric, cumin, ground paprika and tomato paste in a bowl. Then add the salmon fillets and coat. Place on the lined baking tray and bake for 15-20 minutes or until cooked to your liking.

Combine the lettuce, tomatoes, cucumber and red onion in a bowl and set aside.

To make the dressing, add the Greek yoghurt, grated cucumber and lemon juice to a small bowl. Stir to combine and set aside.

When the salmon is cooked, break it apart to make little salmon flakes. Top the salad with the salmon and drizzle with the yoghurt dressing.

**NOTE:**
› Make pickled onions instead by adding the sliced onion to a jar
  with ½ water, ½ vinegar and 1 tsp sugar. Refrigerate for 2-3 hours.

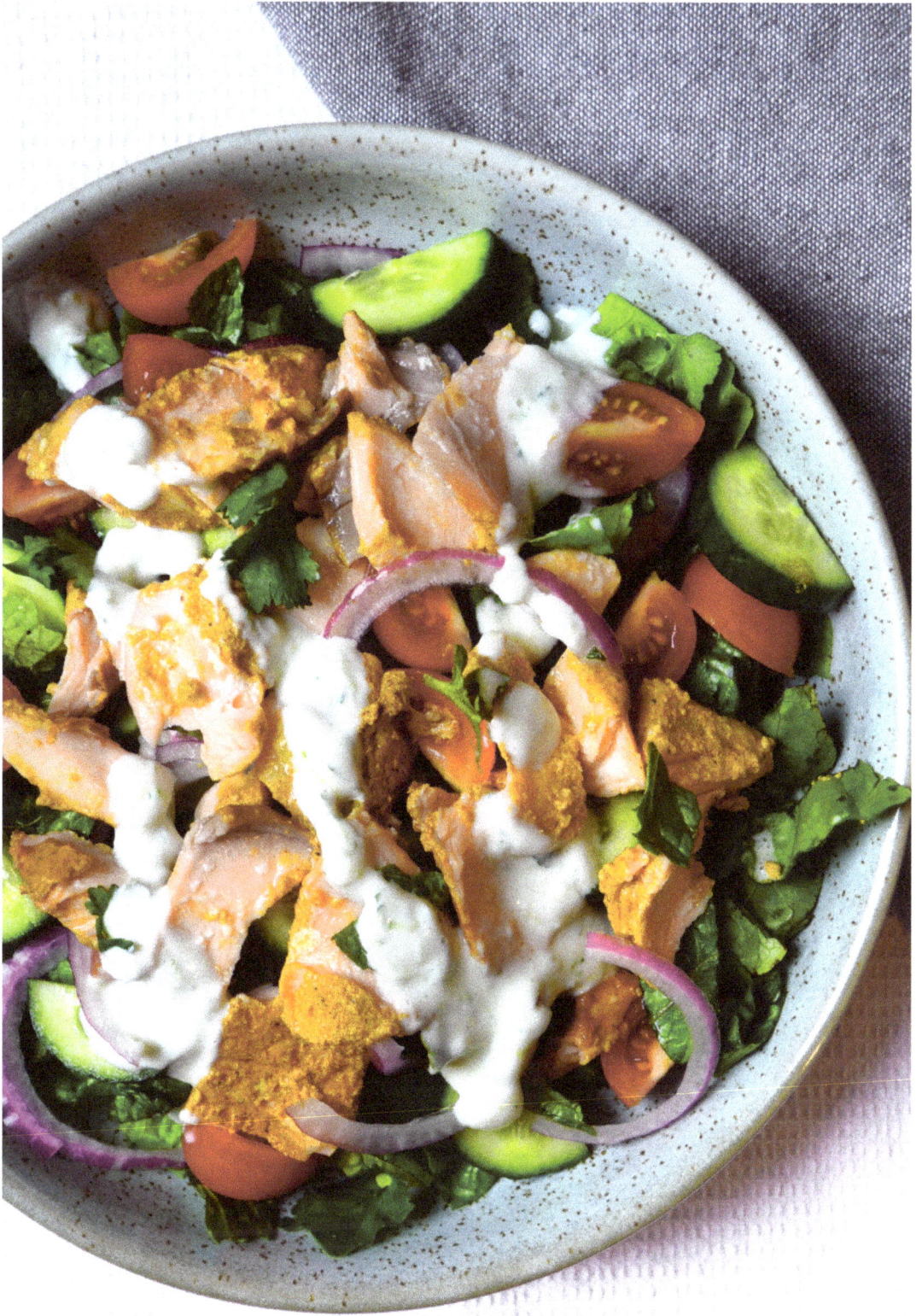

# snacks

Tomato &
Eggplant Dip

Almond
Seed Bar

Chocolate &
Pistachio Slice

Puffed Quinoa &
Berry Slice

Chunky Capsicum
Pesto Dip

Island Dream
Overnight Pudding

# TOMATO & EGGPLANT DIP

**Serves:** 1    **Prep:** 10 minutes    **Cook:** 30 minutes

1 tbsp olive oil
3 garlic cloves, chopped
1 tbsp cumin seeds
1 tbsp coriander seeds
¼ tsp chilli powder
   (optional)
1 eggplant, peeled and
   chopped
3-4 tomatoes, peeled (see
   tip)
¼ coriander bunch,
   chopped
¼ parsley bunch, chopped
1 cup water
1 lemon, juiced
1 tbsp tomato paste

**Serving suggestions:**
Coriander, chopped
Parsley, chopped
Olive oil
Sourdough bread
Crackers
Vegetable sticks

In a pan on medium heat with olive oil, add the chopped garlic, cumin seeds, coriander seeds and chilli powder and sauté for 2-3 minutes until the garlic is soft.

Add the eggplant, tomatoes, coriander, parsley and water to the pan. Simmer for 20 minutes or until the ingredients are soft. Stir often.

Add the lemon juice and tomato paste to the pan and cook for another 5 minutes.

Remove from the heat and allow to cool down before blending until smooth.

If desired, top with some fresh parsley, coriander and a drizzle of olive oil. Serve with crackers, veggie sticks, or sourdough bread. Can be enjoyed warm or cold.

**TIP:**
› To peel the tomatoes easily, score the top of the tomatoes, boil for 15 minutes and then add to ice water for 5 minutes. Peel the skin from the scored section.

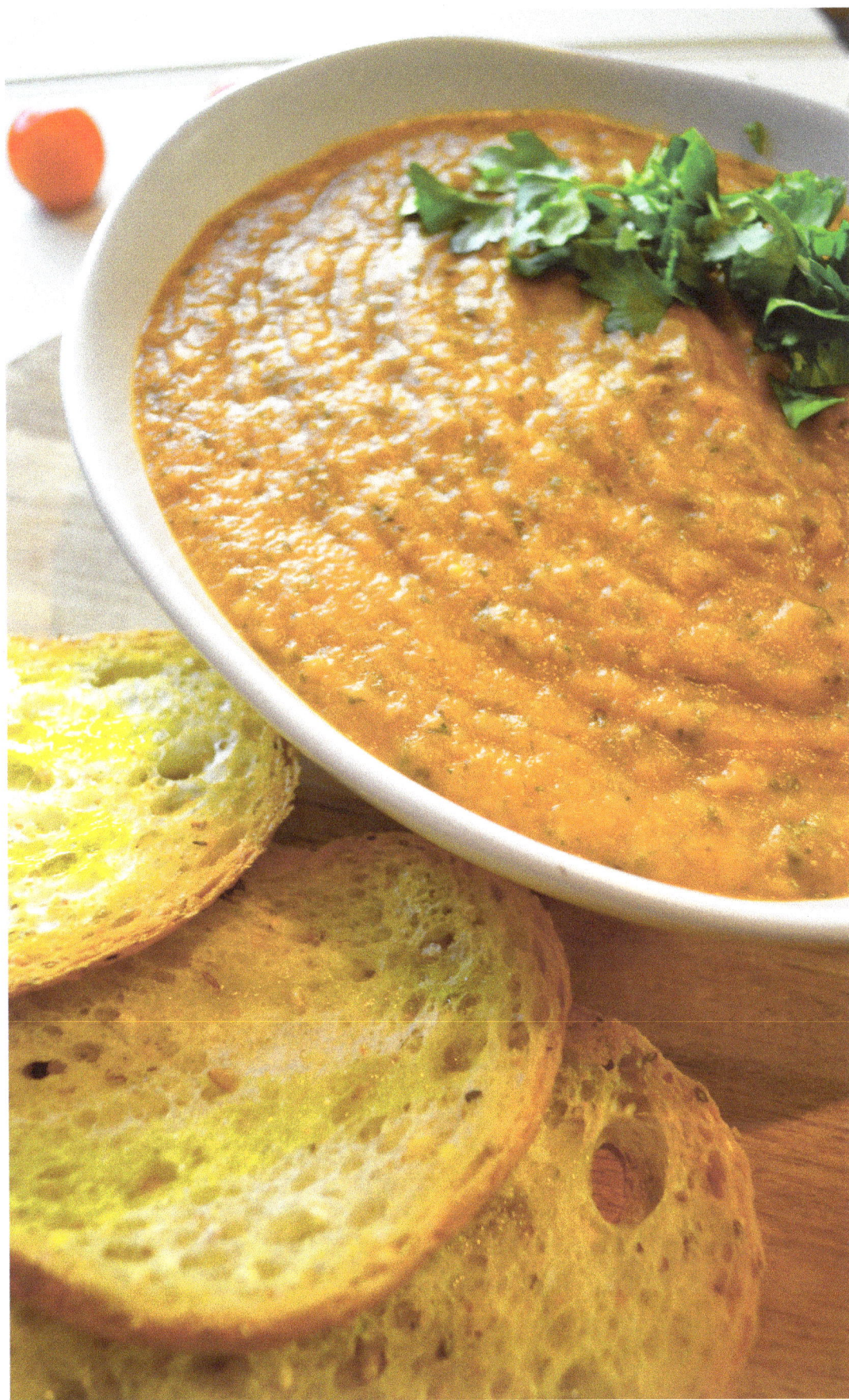

# ALMOND SEED BAR

**Serves:** 6-8 bars    **Prep:** 5 minutes    **Cook:** 30 minutes

1 cup almonds
⅓ cup mixed seeds
  (sunflower, pepita, chia,
  sesame seeds)
4 tbsp malt rice syrup

Preheat the oven to 160°C fan-forced.

In an oven-safe dish, add the almonds and mixed seeds, then dry roast for approximately 10 minutes. Remove from the oven.

Transfer the roasted nuts and seeds into a bowl and stir through the malt rice syrup.

Line a baking dish with parchment paper, add the mixture and press it down evenly.

Bake in the oven for 15-20 minutes.

Remove from the oven and allow it to cool and harden.

Chop into bar-shaped pieces or bite-sized bits.

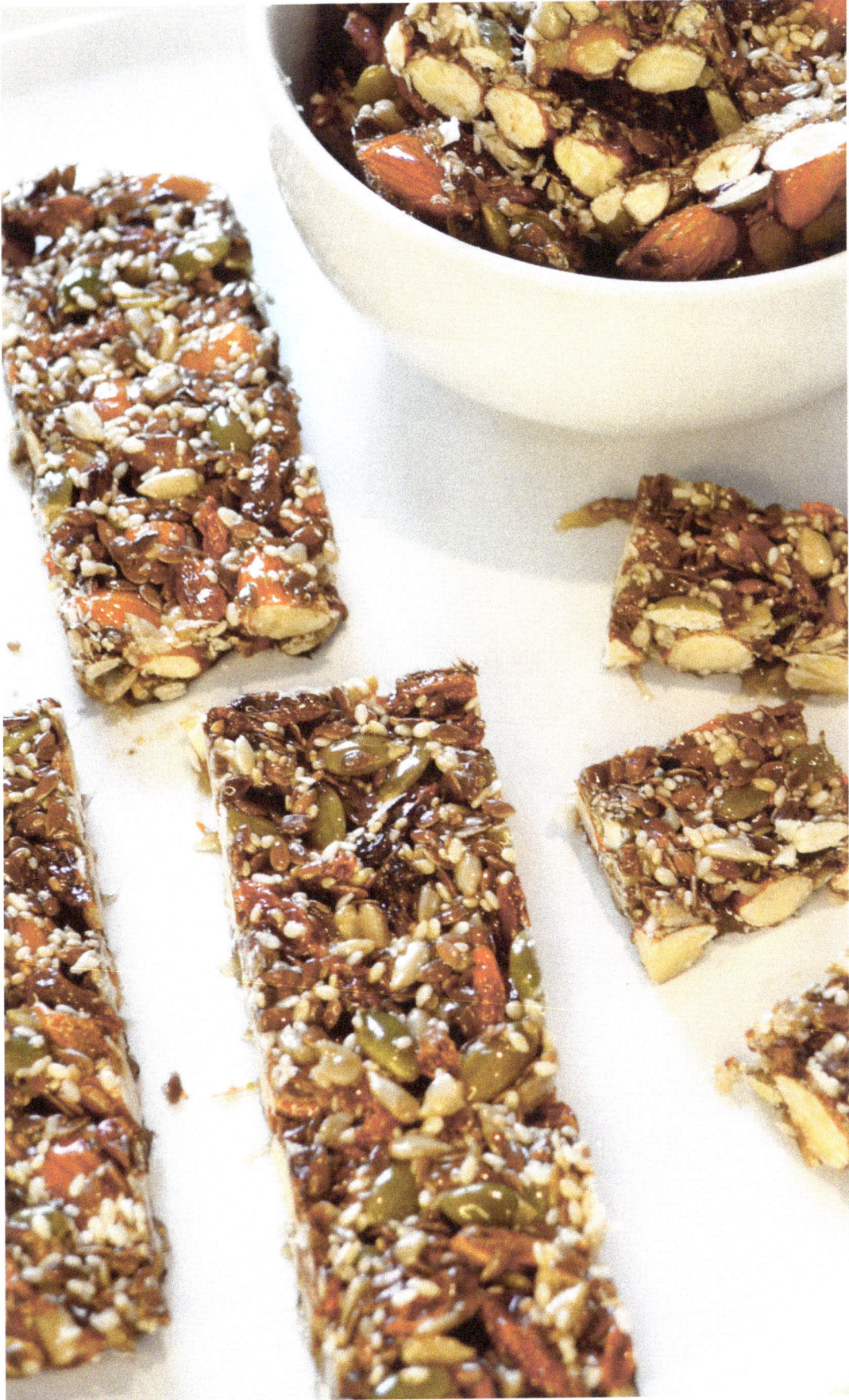

# CHOCOLATE & PISTACHIO SLICE

**Serves:** 12 pieces    **Prep:** 5 minutes    **Cook:** 30 minutes

**For the base:**
6 medjool dates
¾ cup almonds
¼ cup flaxseeds
¼ pepitas seeds
1 tbsp maca powder
   (optional)
1 tbsp chia seeds
¼ cup water

**For the centre:**
1 cup pistachios
1 tbsp water (to loosen
   mixture if needed)
1 tbsp maple syrup
½ cup shredded coconut

**For the topping:**
1 cup dark chocolate
1 tbsp pistachios, roughly
   chopped (optional)

Remove all pistachios from their shells and put the ones for the centre into a bowl of water to soak. Set aside.

To make the base, put the dates, almonds, flaxseed, pepitas, maca powder, chia seeds and water in a food processor. Blend until combined.

In a lined bread tin, transfer the base mixture and press down evenly. Refrigerate for 10 minutes to set.

Once the base has set, drain the pistachios soaking in water. Add to a blender with water and maple syrup and blend until a smooth creamy texture has formed. Add more water if the mixture is too thick. Stir through the shredded coconut.

Remove the base from the refrigerator and cover with the topping. Return to the fridge for another 10 minutes.

Meanwhile, melt the dark chocolate by placing it in a bowl and microwaving in 60-second intervals, taking caution when removing the bowl. Stir in between each interval until the chocolate is completely melted.

Remove the base from the refrigerator and top with melted chocolate and extra pistachios, if desired.

Slice into bars or bites.

Store in an airtight container in the fridge for up to a week.

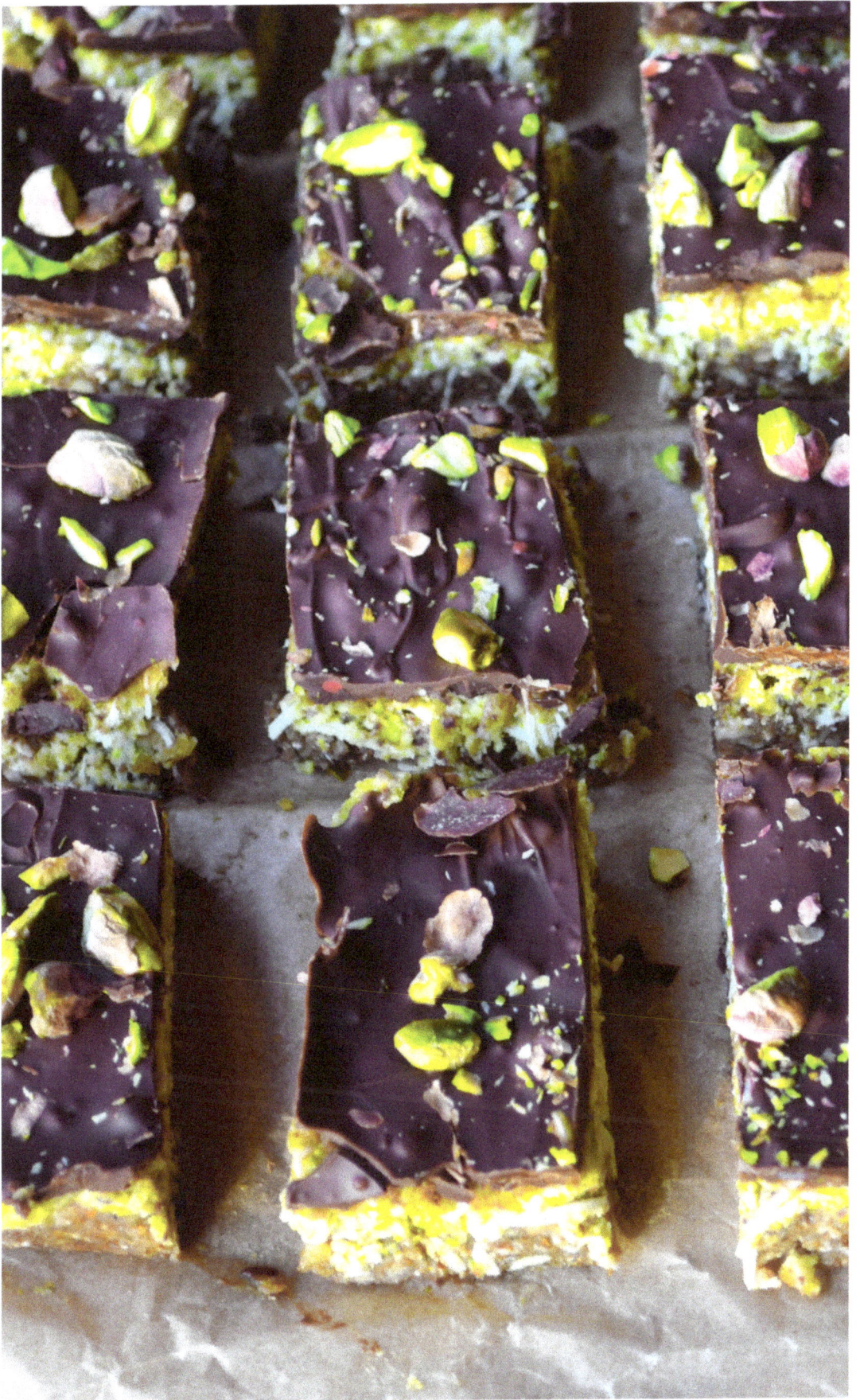

# PUFFED QUINOA & BERRY SLICE

**Serves:** 8 pieces    **Prep:** 5 minutes    **Cook:** 2 hours

2 cups puffed quinoa
½ cup almond butter
½ cup frozen raspberries
  and strawberries
1 heaped tbsp vanilla
  protein powder (optional)
1 tbsp maca powder
2 tbsp water

**Topping (optional):**
1 tbsp almonds, roughly
  chopped
1 tbsp pistachios, roughly
  chopped
1 tbsp shredded or
  desiccated coconut
1 tbsp frozen raspberries,
  crushed

In a mixing bowl, add the puffed quinoa, almond butter, frozen berries, vanilla protein powder (if using), maca powder and water. Combine the ingredients using your hands, ensuring the almond butter coats the puffed quinoa.

Line a bread tin and transfer the mixture, spreading it out evenly. Top with chopped almonds, pistachios, coconut and crushed raspberries, if desired.

Allow to set in the refrigerator for at least 2 hours.

Slice into bitesized pieces or bars. Store in the fridge until ready to eat.

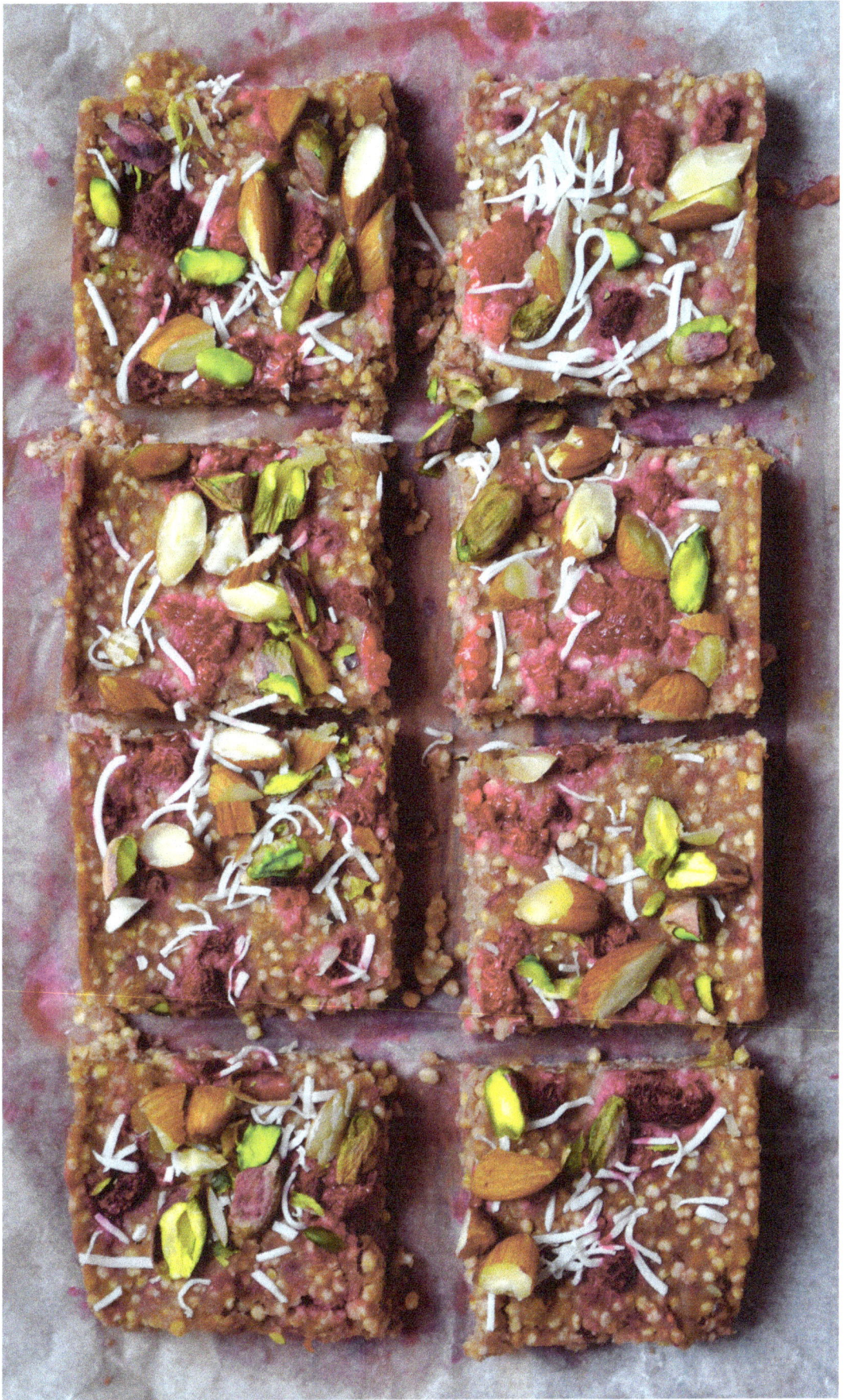

# CHUNKY CAPSICUM PESTO DIP

**Serves:** 1    **Prep:** 5 minutes    **Cook:** 40 minutes

2 large capsicums, halved
  with seeds removed*
⅓ cup cashews, roughly
  chopped
2 tbsp olive oil
1 tbsp lemon juice
1 tbsp white wine vinegar
Salt and pepper to taste

Pre-heat the oven to 200°C fan-forced.

Roast the capsicum for 25-30 minutes until the skin has charred. Remove from oven and allow to cool before peeling the skin off the capsicum. Finely chop the rest of the capsicum.

In a bowl, combine the capsicum, cashews, olive oil, lemon juice, vinegar, salt and pepper.

Serve with crackers or veggie sticks.

**NOTE:**
› Alternatively you can use jarred roasted capsicums/peppers in brine to reduce cooking time.

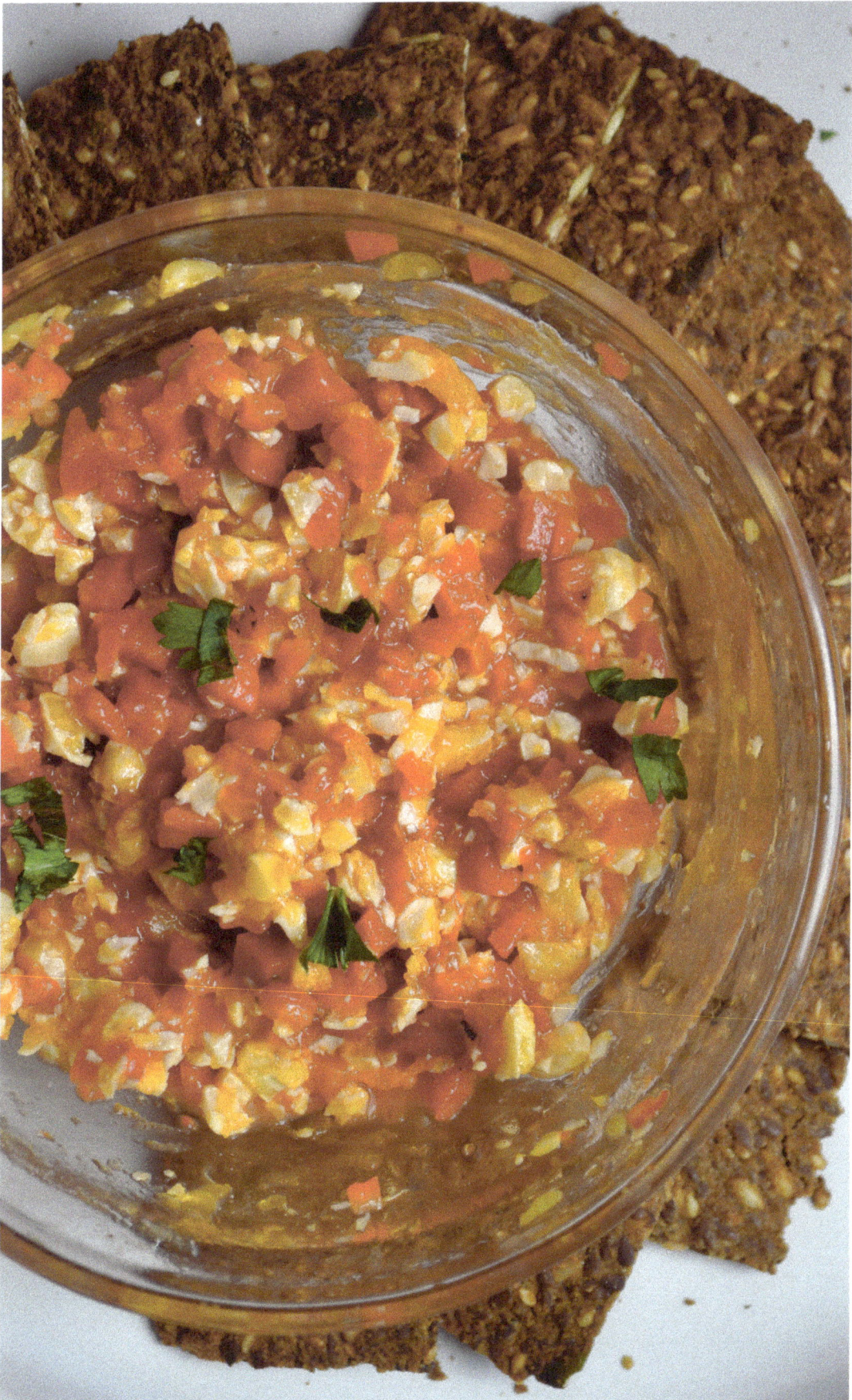

# ISLAND DREAM OVERNIGHT PUDDING

**Serves:** 2    **Prep:** 5 minutes    **Cook:** 2-3 hours/overnight

**For the oats:**
1 ¼ cup oats
3 tbsp chia seeds
2 heaped tbsp vanilla or
   plain protein powder
2 cups water

**For the sauce:**
1 tbsp coconut oil
2 tbsp almond butter
¼ cup canned coconut milk
1 tbsp shredded coconut

In a food processor, add the oats, chia seeds and protein powder. Blend until the oats have become a fine powder. Add to a glass container and combine with the water. Refrigerate for 20 minutes to allow the water to absorb.

In a small saucepan, add the coconut oil and almond butter and stir continuously until the butter and oil have melted. Then stir through the coconut milk until well combined. Remove from heat and allow to cool.

Divide the oat mixture into 2 bowls or dishes. Top the oats with the coconut almond sauce and garnish with the shredded coconut. Refrigerate for another 2-3 hours or overnight.

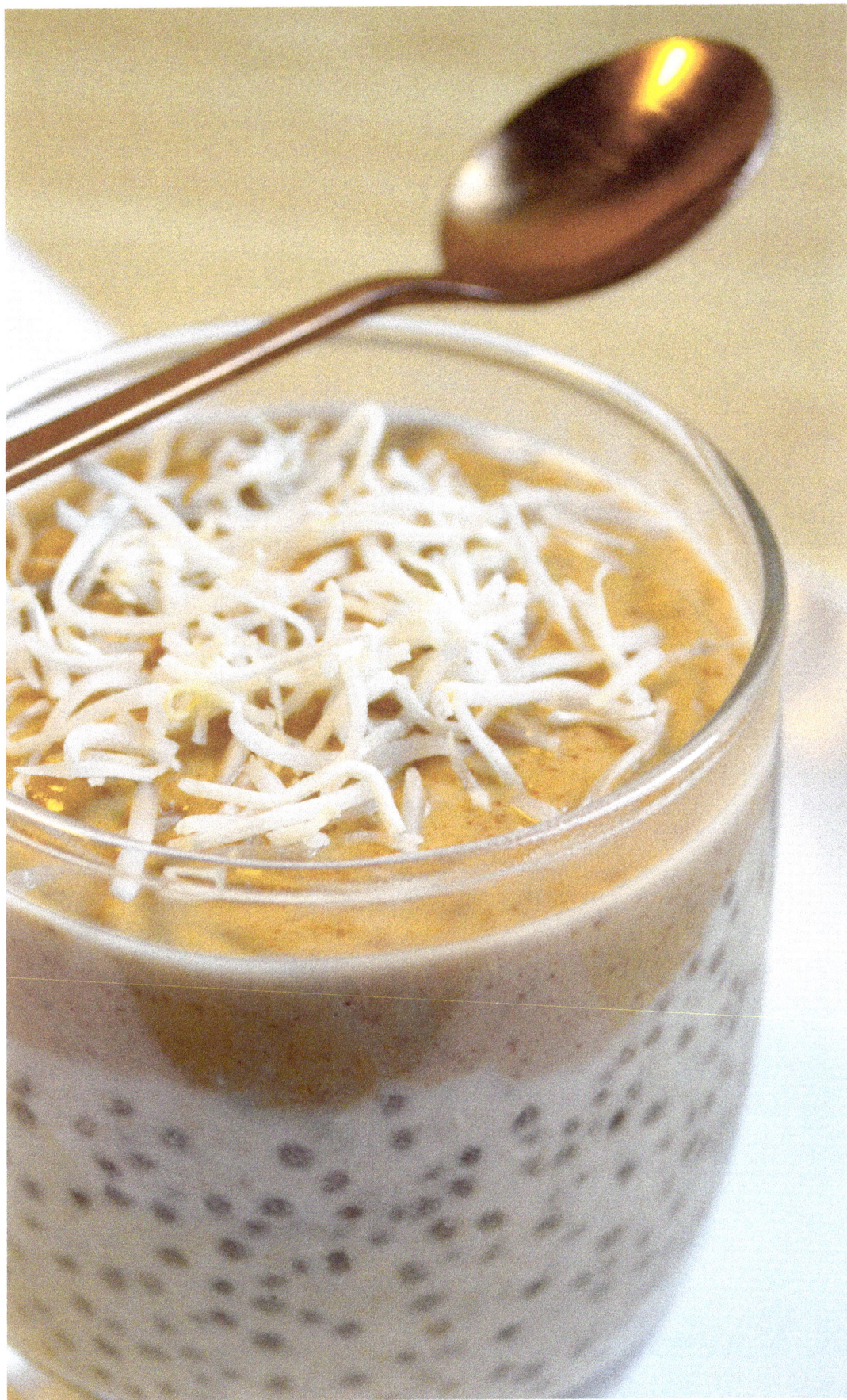

luteal

phase

# HERO FOODS

## NUTRIENTS FOR THE LUTEAL PHASE
ZINC | CALCIUM | IRON | MAGNESIUM | B-VITAMINS

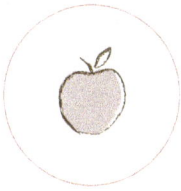

APPLE

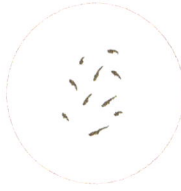

BROWN RICE

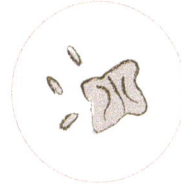

NUTS
(PINE & WALNUTS)

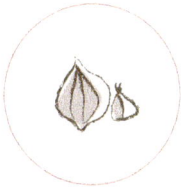

ONION & GARLIC

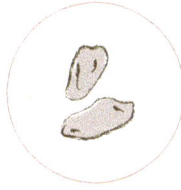

DATES & RAISINS

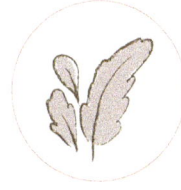

LEAFY GREENS

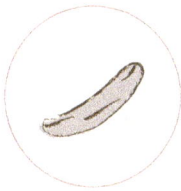

CUCUMBER

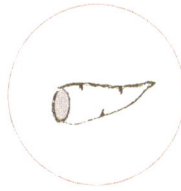

SWEET POTATO

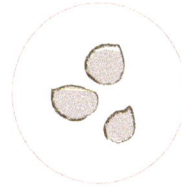

CHICKPEAS

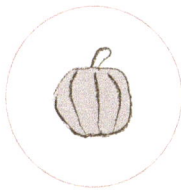

PUMPKIN

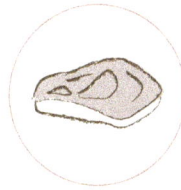

BEEF & TURKEY

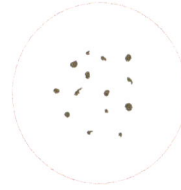

SEEDS

luteal
recipes

# breakfast

Balance &
Calm Smoothie

Spiced Sweet
Potato Pie Oats

Deconstructed
Bubble & Squeak

Sweet Potato &
Leek Breakfast Hash

Pear Pancake Bowls

Pumpkin &
Onion Frittata

Creamy Oatmeal
with Poached Pears

# BALANCE & CALM SMOOTHIE

**Serves:** 1    **Prep:** 5 minutes    **Cook:** N/A

½ frozen banana
1 cup sweet potato or
  pumpkin, steamed
1 tbsp tahini
1 tbsp flaxseed meal
1 tsp cinnamon
1 tsp nutmeg
1 tsp ginger
1 tbsp sunflower seeds
1 tsp raw honey
1 cup water
1 heaped tbsp protein
  powder
1 tsp cacao

Add all the ingredients to a blender and blend until smooth.
Serve immediately.

*This recipe also doubles as a snack option.*

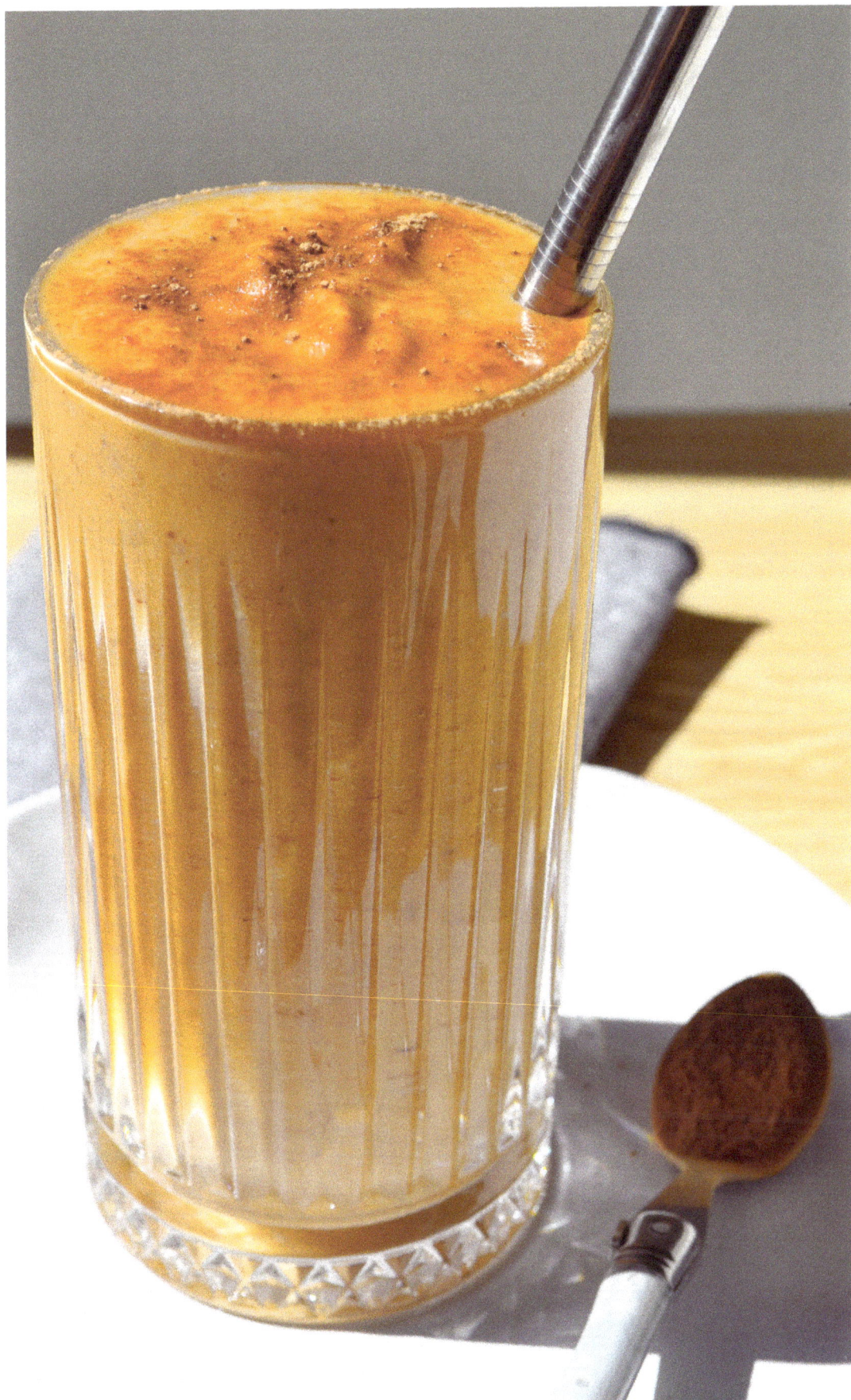

# SPICED SWEET POTATO PIE OATS

**Serves:** 4    **Prep:** 10 minutes    **Cook:** 20 minutes

1 sweet potato, peeled and diced
1 pear, peeled and diced
2 cups oats
2 tbsp vanilla protein powder
1 tbsp tahini
¼ cup chia seeds
1 tsp cinnamon
1 tsp nutmeg
300ml coconut milk

**To serve:**
140g Greek yoghurt (per serve)
Pinch of cinnamon or nutmeg

Preheat the oven to 180°C.

In a steamer or steaming basket over a pot of boiling water, add the sweet potato and pear. Steam for 5-10 minutes or until the potato and pear are soft.

In a blender, add the steamed sweet potato and pear, along with the oats, protein powder, tahini, chia seeds, cinnamon, nutmeg and coconut milk. Blend until smooth. Transfer mixture to a 20x20cm baking tray and smooth the surface.

Bake in the oven for 15 minutes or until the oats are golden brown.

Serve with Greek yoghurt and a pinch of cinnamon or nutmeg if desired.

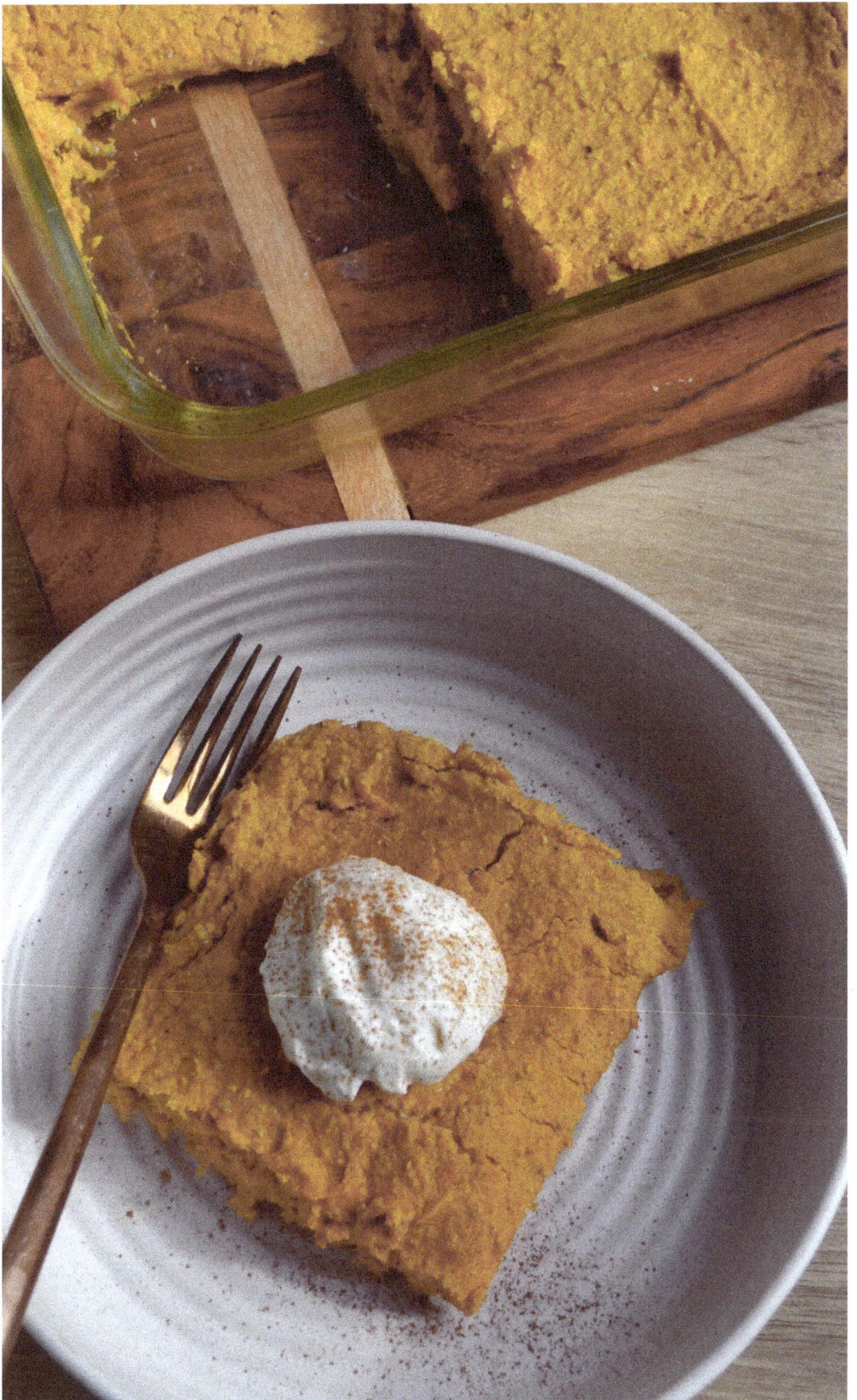

# DECONSTRUCTED BUBBLE & SQUEAK

**Serves:** 4     **Prep:** 10 minutes     **Cook:** 25 minutes

1 sweet potato, peeled and diced
1 carrot, halved lengthwise and sliced
1 tsp olive oil
400g turkey breast slices, diced
¼ of a medium-sized white cabbage, thinly sliced
1 leek, sliced
1 head broccoli, cut into small florets
4 eggs, boiled (1 per serve)
¼ cup kalamata olives, sliced
1 cup of spinach leaves, chopped
1 tbsp caraway seeds
Salt and pepper, to season

**To serve:**
Lemon wedges (optional)

Steam the diced sweet potato and sliced carrot for 5-10 minutes until tender.

In the meantime, add the olive oil and diced turkey to a pan on medium heat. Lightly brown for 2 minutes, then remove from the pan.

In the same pan, add the sliced cabbage and sauté for 10 minutes. Add the sliced leek and continue to sauté for a further 5 minutes.

Then add the broccoli florets, sweet potato and carrots. Continue to sauté until all vegetables are tender.

In the meantime, boil the eggs for 6 minutes (for a soft-boiled egg), 7 minutes (for a semi-soft-boiled egg), or to your preference. Place the boiled eggs in a bowl of iced water and peel off the shell.

Stir through the kalamata olives, spinach leaves and caraway seeds into the frypan. Season with salt and pepper.

Divide the mixture evenly between 4 plates. Top each serving with a boiled egg and serve with lemon wedges, if desired.

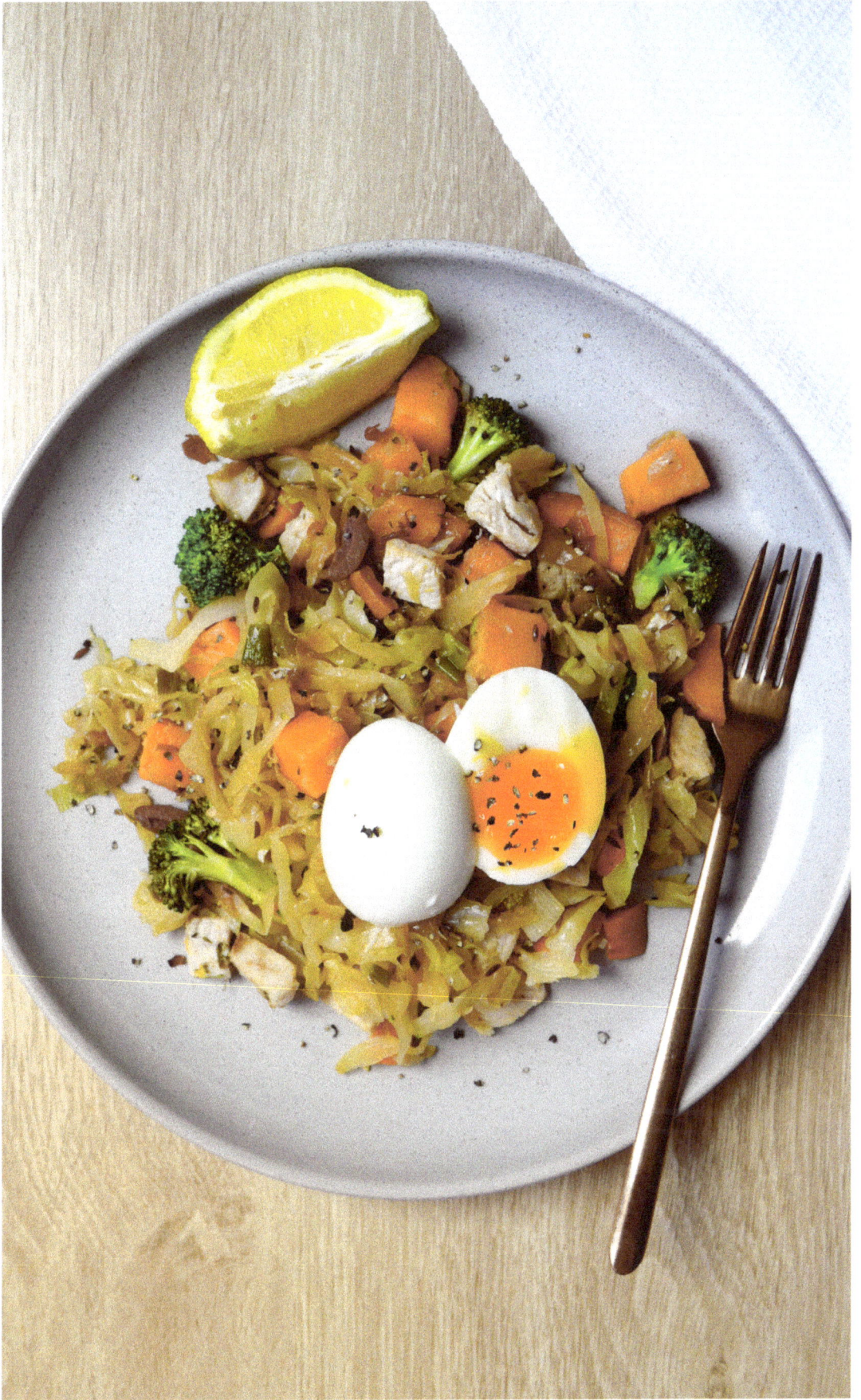

# SWEET POTATO & LEEK BREAKFAST HASH

**Serves:** 4     **Prep:** 10 minutes     **Cook:** 40 minutes

1 tbsp olive oil
1 sweet potato, peeled and
  diced
1 leek, finely sliced
2 capsicums, diced
400g canned diced
  tomatoes
2 cups spinach, chopped
¼ tsp garlic powder
¼ tsp ginger powder
½ tsp sweet paprika
½ tsp cumin
Pinch of salt and pepper
4 eggs

Preheat the oven to 180°C fan-forced.

In a heated oven-proof pan on medium, add the olive oil and diced sweet potato. Allow it to cook until softened, stirring regularly.

Once the potato is tender, add the leek and capsicum to the pan and cook for 4-5 minutes until softened.

Add the diced tomatoes, spinach, garlic powder, ginger powder, paprika and cumin. Season with salt and pepper. Stir to combine.

Create four wells in the mixture and crack an egg into each well. Bake in the oven until the eggs are cooked to your liking.

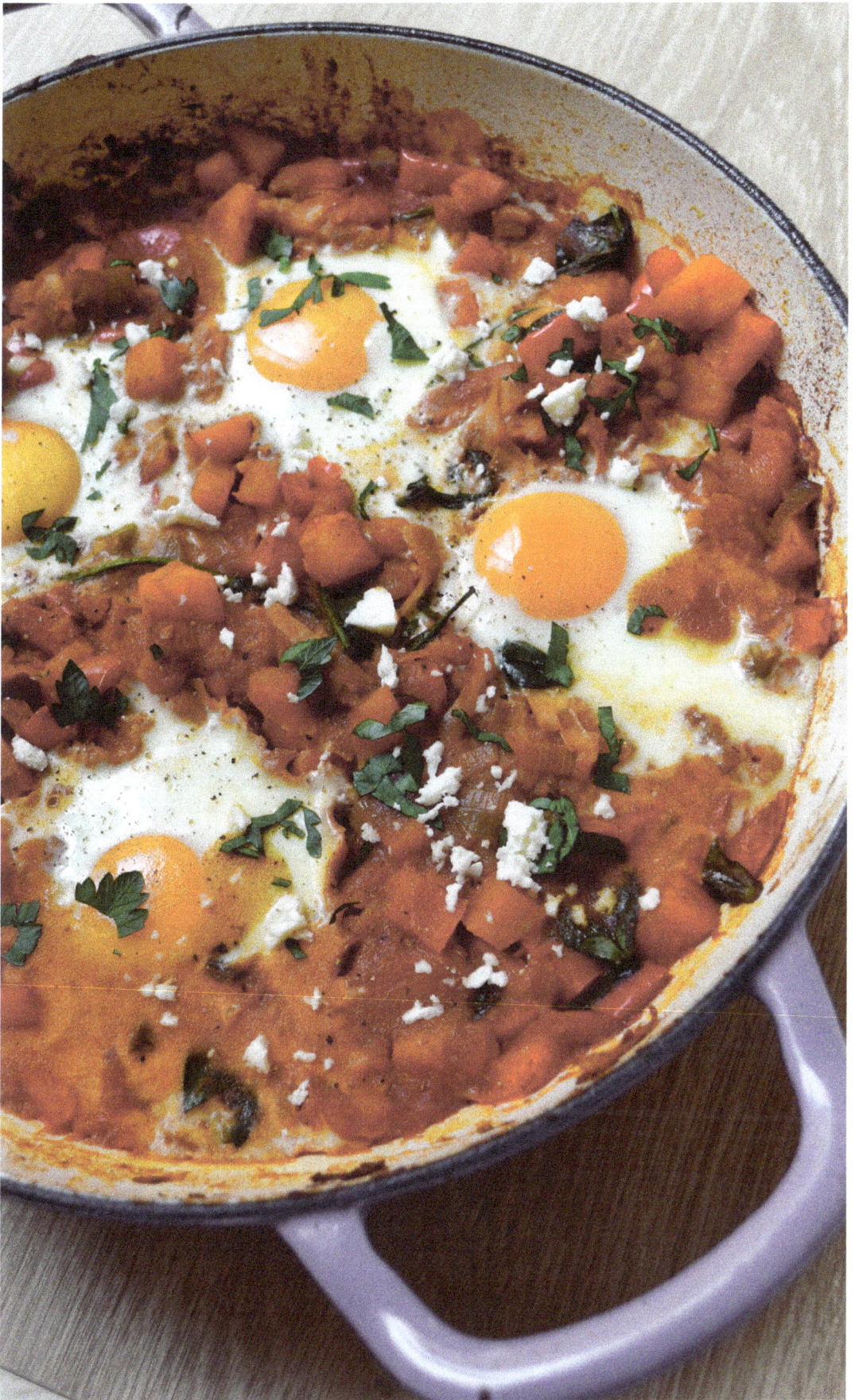

# PEAR PANCAKE BOWLS

**Serves:** 2     **Prep:** 10 minutes     **Cook:** 20 minutes

1 cup rolled oats
1 cup milk of choice
1 tbsp cinnamon
1 tsp baking soda
1 tbsp protein powder
1 pear, peeled and grated

**For the poached fruit:**
1 apple, peeled and diced
1 pear, peeled and diced
1 tsp cinnamon
¼ cup water
¼ tsp vanilla extract

**To serve:**
1 cup Greek Yoghurt
2 tbsp crushed walnuts
2 tbsp sunflower seeds
2 tbsp pepita seeds
Maple syrup (optional)

Preheat the oven to 180°C fan-forced.

In a food processor, blend the rolled oats to make oat flour. Add the milk, cinnamon, baking soda and protein powder, then blend again until smooth. Stir in the grated pear.

Transfer the mixture to 2 single-serve glass baking dishes and bake in the oven for 20 minutes or until slightly firm and lightly golden on top.

Meanwhile, make the poached fruit by adding the apple, pear, cinnamon, water and vanilla extract to a pot heated on medium. Cover with a lid and allow to cook for 10 minutes or until tender.

Serve the baked pear pancake bowls with the Greek yoghurt and top with the poached fruit, walnuts, sunflower seeds and pepita seeds. Drizzle with maple syrup, if desired.

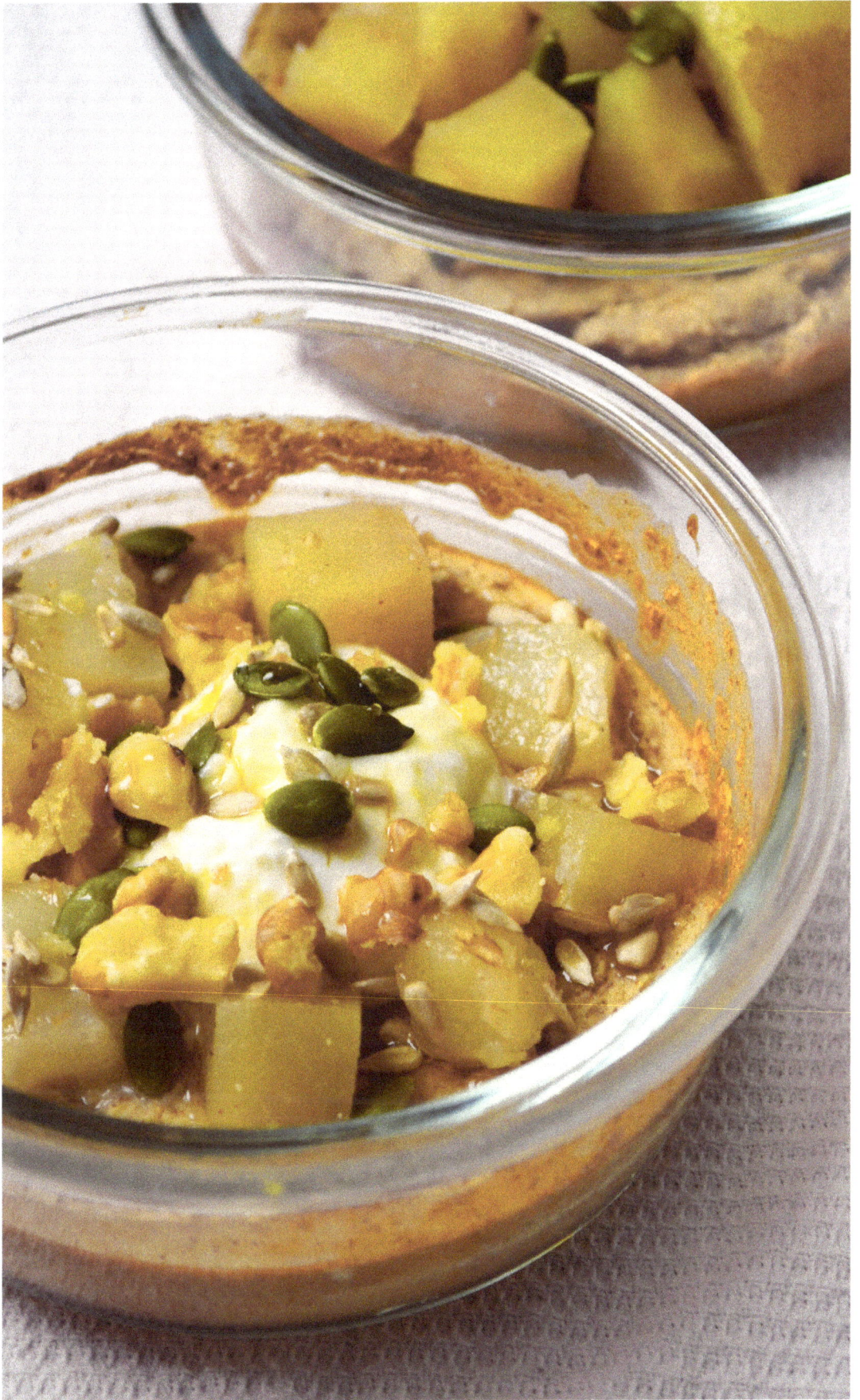

# PUMPKIN & ONION FRITTATA

**Serves:** 4     **Prep:** 10 minutes     **Cook:** 40 minutes

2 cups butternut pumpkin, peeled and diced
Olive oil
1 red onion, finely sliced
1 cup spinach, roughly chopped
8 eggs
¾ cup cottage cheese
2 tbsp hemp seeds
1 tbsp dried thyme
¼ cup milk
⅓ cup chopped herbs (like parsley and dill)
Salt and pepper
⅓ cup feta, crumbled

To serve:
Avocado

Preheat the oven to 180°C fan-forced.

Using a steaming basket, steam the diced pumpkin until tender.

In a fry pan on medium heat, add a drizzle of olive oil and add the red onion. Sauté until softened. Add the steamed pumpkin and spinach and cook until the spinach has wilted.

In a bowl, combine the eggs, cottage cheese, hemp seeds, dried thyme, milk, herbs, salt and pepper. Mix well to combine.

In a lined or greased baking dish, add the pumpkin mix and then top with the egg mixture. Stir to combine the ingredients and to mix the hemp seeds evenly (as they can clump). Top with the feta cheese and bake in the oven for about 30 minutes.

Remove from the oven and serve with avocado if desired.

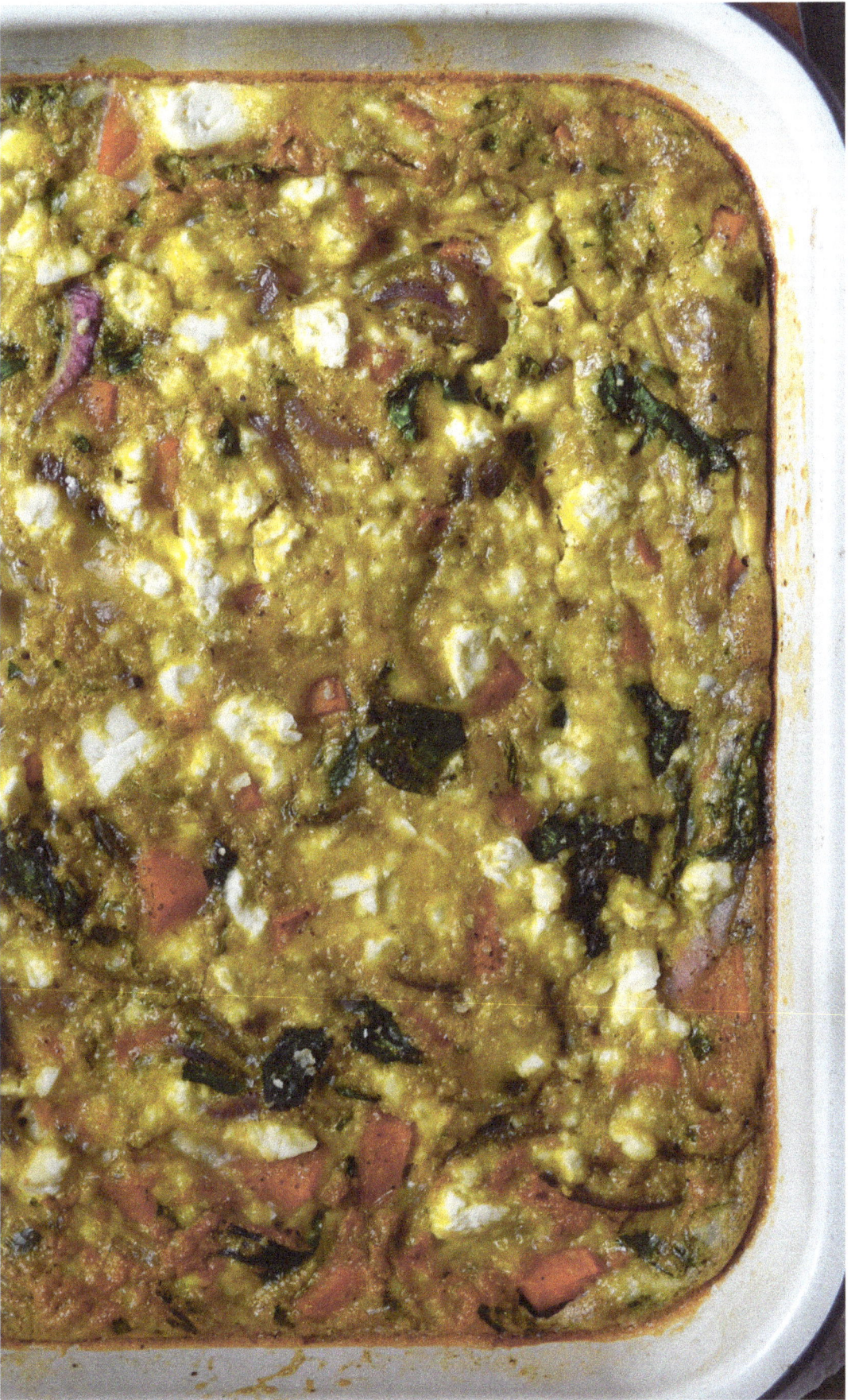

# CREAMY OATMEAL
## WITH POACHED PEARS

**Serves:** 4     **Prep:** 5 minutes     **Cook:** 10 minutes

1 ½ cup oats
¼ cup chia seeds
1 tbsp flaxseed meal
1 tsp cinnamon
1 cup milk of choice
2 cups water
1 tbsp maple syrup

**For the poached pears**
4 pears, peeled
1 tsp cinnamon

**To serve:**
3 tbsp Greek yoghurt
1 tbsp pepitas
1 tbsp sunflower seeds
Maple syrup (optional)
Cinnamon (optional)

In a saucepan filled with the water, add the pears and cinnamon. Poach on a medium heat for about 10 minutes or until the pears can be easily pierced with a knife. Remove from water, slice the pears and set aside.

In a food processor, add the oats, chia seeds, flaxseed meal and cinnamon. Blend until a fine consistency has been made.

Add the oat mixture to a saucepan. Combine the milk and water and simmer over a low heat for 5 minutes. If the porridge gets too thick, add more water to reach your preferred consistency.

Serve into bowls or containers and top with the poached pears, Greek yoghurt, pepitas, sunflower seeds, a sprinkle of cinnamon and a drizzle of maple syrup if desired.

**NOTE:**
› If meal prepping, add an additional 2 tbsp of water or milk before reheating to loosen the porridge as the flaxseed will cause it to thicken when refrigerated.

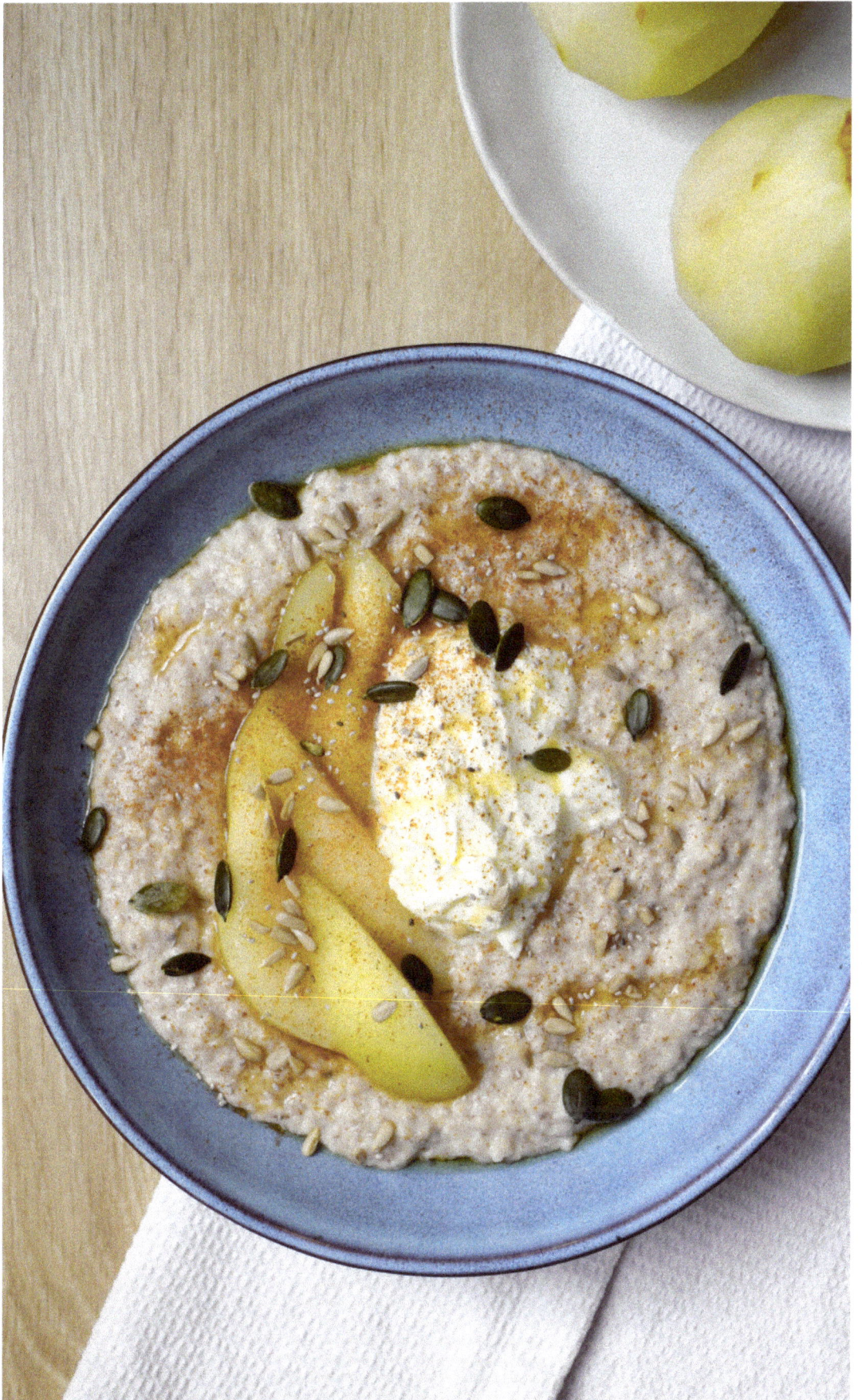

# mains

Beef & Slaw Taco
Nourish Bowl

Sweet Potato Falafel
Nourish Bowl

Golden Chicken &
Mung Bean Soup

Autumn Salad
with Tahini Maple Dressing

Root Veggie Soup

Turkey Patties
with Roast Veggies
and Quinoa

Cauliflower &
Leek Soup

Deconstructed
Sushi Bowls

Creamy Chickpea &
Sweet Potato Curry

Turkey & Roasted
Veggie Tray Bake

# BEEF & SLAW TACO NOURISH BOWL

**Serves:** 4     **Prep:** 15 minutes     **Cook:** 15 minutes

1 tsp olive oil
1 garlic clove, chopped
500g beef mince
1 tbsp cumin
½ tbsp sweet paprika
½ tbsp dried oregano
¼ tsp chilli powder
½ tsp garlic powder
2 tbsp tomato paste
2 tbsp water
¼ purple cabbage, grated
¼ white cabbage, grated
1 carrot, grated
1 cucumber, sliced
Brown rice, cooked

**For the guac sauce:**
1 avocado
1 lime, juiced
¼ cup coriander
1 tbsp olive oil

In a pan on medium heat with olive oil, add the garlic and sauté for 1 minute.

Add the beef mince, breaking it up with a spoon and cook until browned. Add cumin, paprika, oregano, chilli powder and garlic powder to the mince, stirring to combine.

Add the tomato paste and water, stirring through until combined and thickened.

Meanwhile, make the slaw by adding the grated carrot and cabbage to a bowl.

In a food processor, add the avocado, lime juice, coriander and olive oil. Blend until smooth and then add half to the cabbage mixture.

Serve in a bowl with the rice, topping with the beef, slaw, cucumber and remaining guac.

**NOTE:**
› You can also serve this as tacos, by substituting the rice out for tortillas of choice.

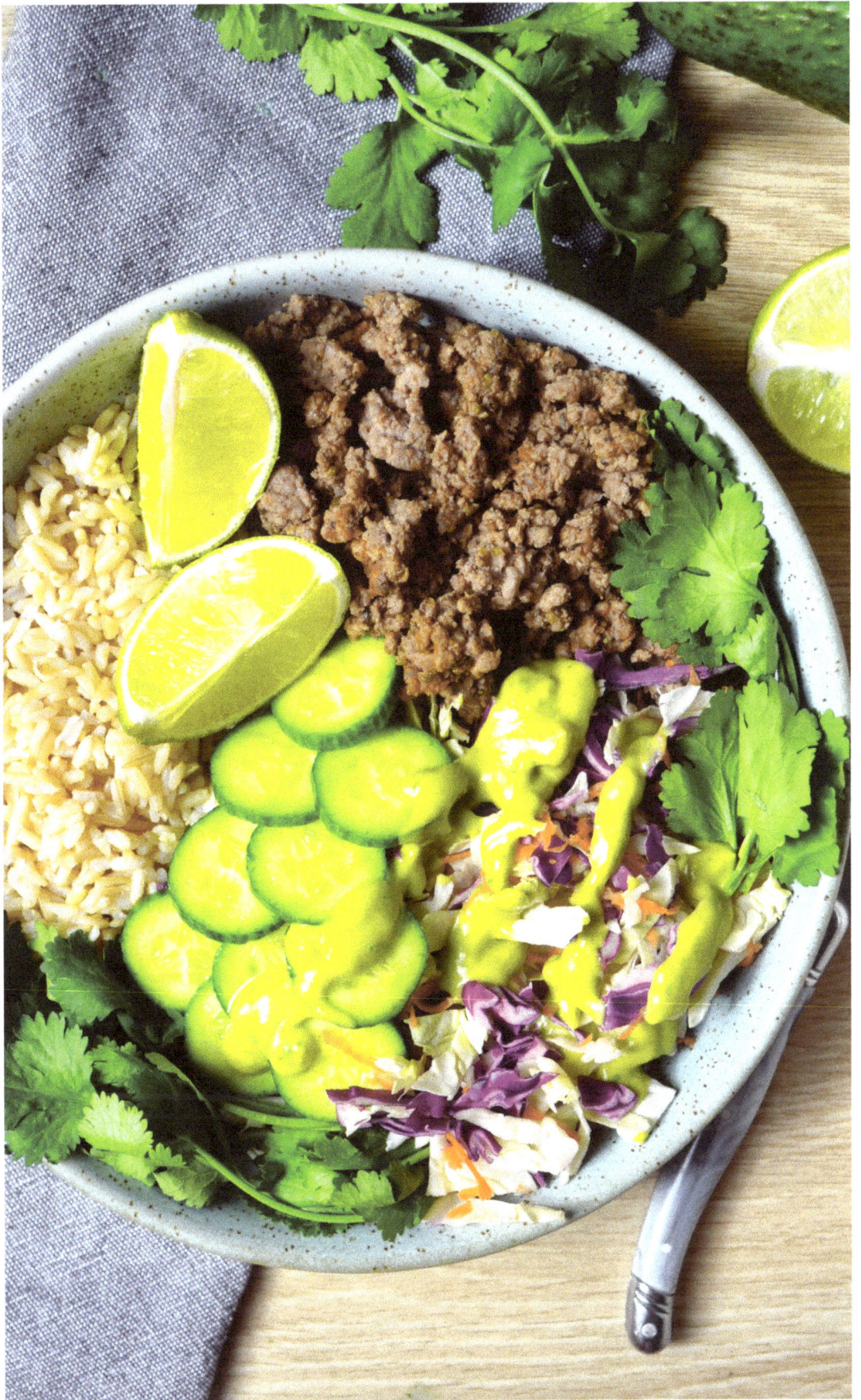

# SWEET POTATO FALAFEL NOURISH BOWL

**Serves:** 4    **Prep:** 10 minutes    **Cook:** 60 minutes

**For the falafel:**
400g chickpeas
¼ sweet potato
1 tightly packed cup mixed
  green herbs (mint, parsley,
  coriander)
1 red onion
1 garlic clove
1 tsp ground cumin
1 tsp ground coriander
1 tbsp chickpea flour
Olive oil spray

**For the bowl:**
¾ sweet potato, roasted
3 cups spinach, roughly
  chopped
½ cup mint, roughly
  chopped
2 tomatoes, diced
2 cucumbers, diced
½ cup kalamata olives
Roasted chickpeas (see
  page 233)
Hummus dip (see page 231)

Preheat the oven to 190°C fan-forced and line a baking tray.

Place all of the sweet potato (for the falafel and the bowl) onto the baking tray and bake in the oven for 20 minutes. Remove once softened.

To make the falafel, add the chickpeas, ¼ of the baked sweet potato, herbs, onion, garlic, cumin, coriander and chickpea flour into a food processor and blend until combined.

Replace the baking paper on the tray and lightly coat it with olive oil. With damp hands, roll the falafel mix into balls and place onto the tray. Spray the falafels with more olive oil. Bake for approximately 30-40 minutes or until browned, turning halfway through.

To serve, construct the bowl with all the falafel and remaining ingredients.

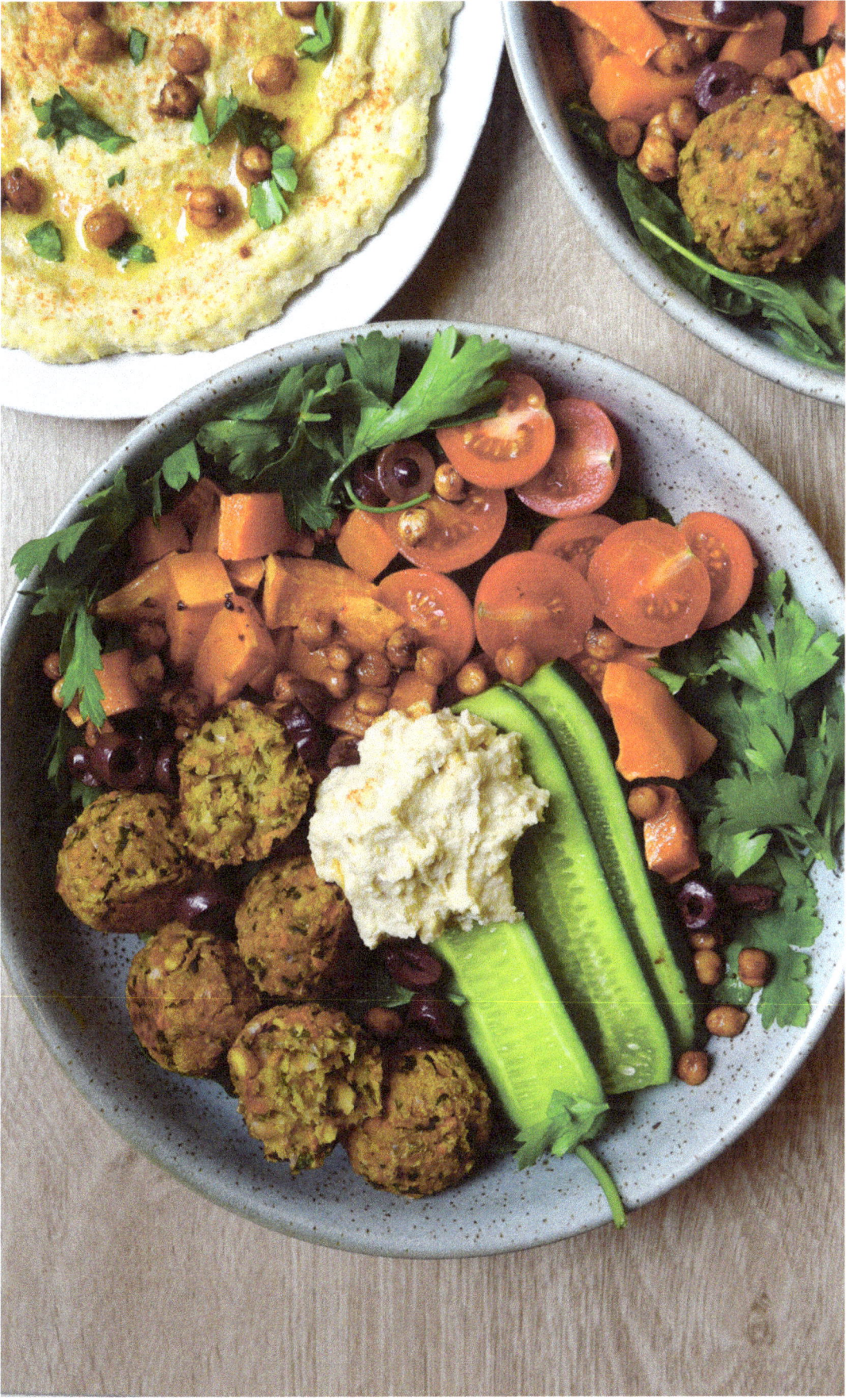

# GOLDEN CHICKEN & MUNG BEAN SOUP

**Serves:** 4   **Prep:** 10 minutes   **Cook:** 45 minutes

1 leek, finely sliced
4 spring onions, chopped (whites and greens separated)
1 cup dried mung beans
1 white onion, halved
4 garlic cloves
4 tbsp fresh ginger, chopped
2 celery stalks, chopped
1 carrot, chopped
6 cups chicken bone broth (see page 245)
500g cooked shredded chicken
1 cup baby spinach
1 tbsp ground turmeric
Salt and pepper, to taste

Heat a drizzle of olive oil in a large pot over medium heat. Add the leek and the white parts of the spring onion. Sauté for 3–5 minutes until softened and fragrant. Remove from the pot and set aside.

To the same pot, add the mung beans, white onion, garlic, ginger, celery, carrot, and half of the bone broth (about 3 cups). Bring to a boil, then reduce heat and simmer for 30 minutes, or until the mung beans are tender.

Carefully transfer the cooked mixture to a blender and blend until smooth and creamy. (Alternatively, use a stick blender in the pot.)

Return the blended mixture to the pot. Add the remaining bone broth, shredded chicken, spinach, turmeric, the green parts of the spring onion and the sautéed leeks and onion whites. Season with salt and pepper to taste.

Simmer gently for another 10 minutes until the spinach is wilted and everything is warmed through. Add more broth or water if you prefer a thinner consistency.

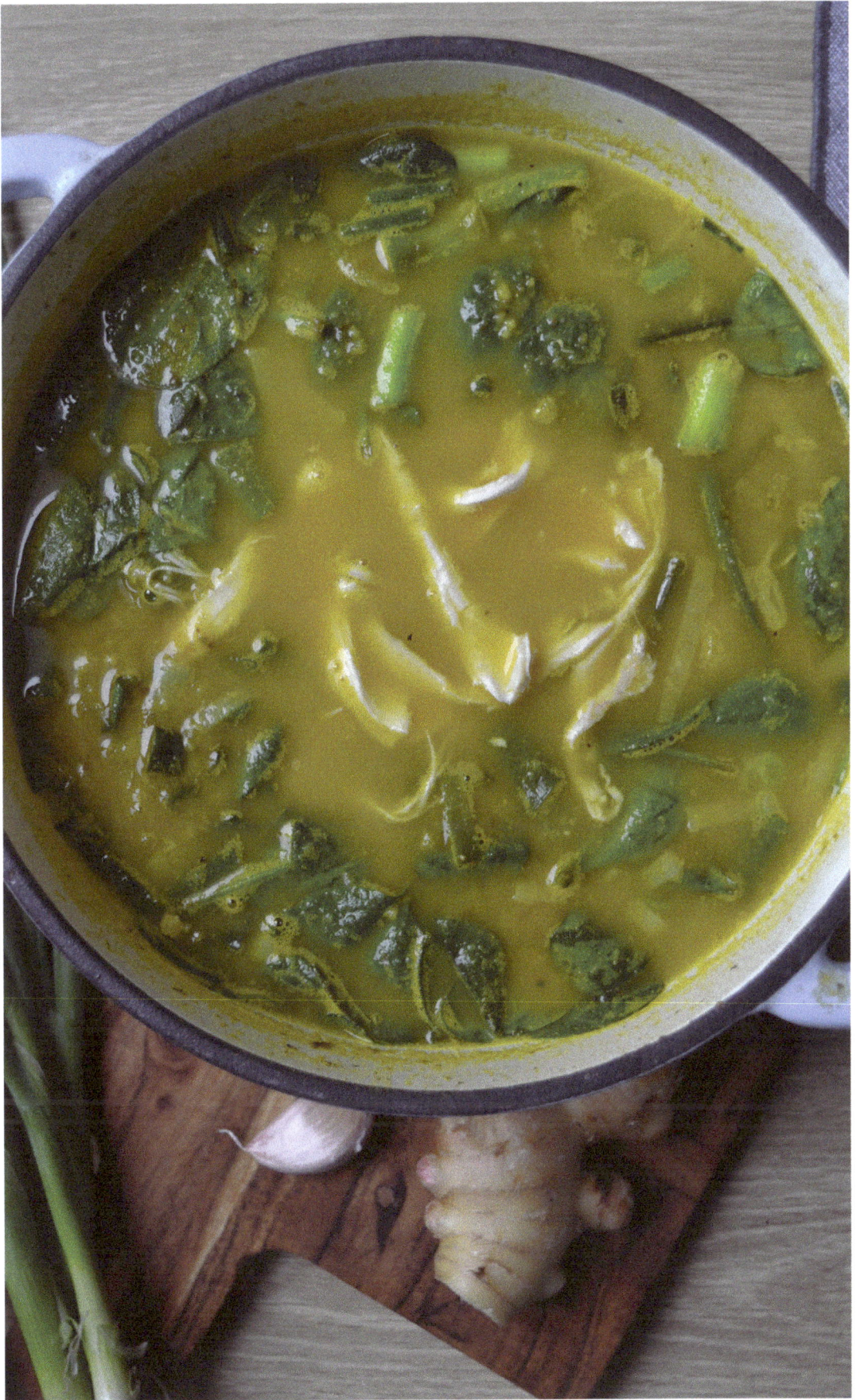

# AUTUMN SALAD
## WITH TAHINI MAPLE DRESSING

**Serves:** 4     **Prep:** 10 minutes     **Cook:** 60 minutes

**For the crispy rice:**
2 cups brown rice, cooked
1 tbsp tamari/soy sauce
1 tsp sesame oil
1 garlic clove, grated

**For the salad:**
1 large sweet potato,
  peeled and diced
Olive oil
1 tsp smoked paprika
Salt and pepper
400g turkey breast
400g chickpeas, drained
  and rinsed
1 bunch Tuscan kale,
  chopped
3 red apples, diced
1 red onion, finely diced
½ cup walnuts, roughly
  chopped
¼ cup dried cranberries/
  raisins, roughly chopped

**For the dressing:**
2 tbsp tahini
1 tbsp olive oil
1 tbsp maple syrup
1 tsp apple cider vinegar
1 tsp Dijon mustard
2–3 tbsp water (adjust for
  preferred consistency)
Salt and pepper

Preheat the oven to 180°C fan-forced.

In a bowl, add the cooked brown rice, tamari/soy sauce, sesame oil and grated garlic and stir to coat the rice evenly. Transfer to a lined baking tray and spread out evenly in a thin layer. Bake for 50–60 minutes until golden and crispy, stirring halfway through.

On a lined baking tray, add the sweet potato and chickpeas. Drizzle with olive oil and season with smoked paprika, salt and pepper. Bake in the oven for 40 minutes.

Heat a pan over medium heat with olive oil and pan fry the turkey breasts. Cook for about 4-5 minutes on each side until cooked through. Set aside and roughly chop into smaller pieces.

In a jar, combine the tahini, olive oil, maple syrup, apple cider vinegar, Dijon mustard, water and salt and pepper. Set aside.

In a large bowl, add the chopped kale. Drizzle with a little olive oil and massage the kale with your hands to make the leaves tender. Then add the apple, red onion, walnuts and cranberries. Add the turkey pieces, sweet potato, chickpeas and crispy rice.

When ready to serve, toss through the dressing and coat the salad evenly.

**NOTE:**
› If meal prepping, keep the kale, apple, onion and walnuts together. If desired, keep the turkey and sweet potato together to warm them up before serving, but they are just as delicious cold. Keep the chickpeas and brown rice separate to stay crispy.

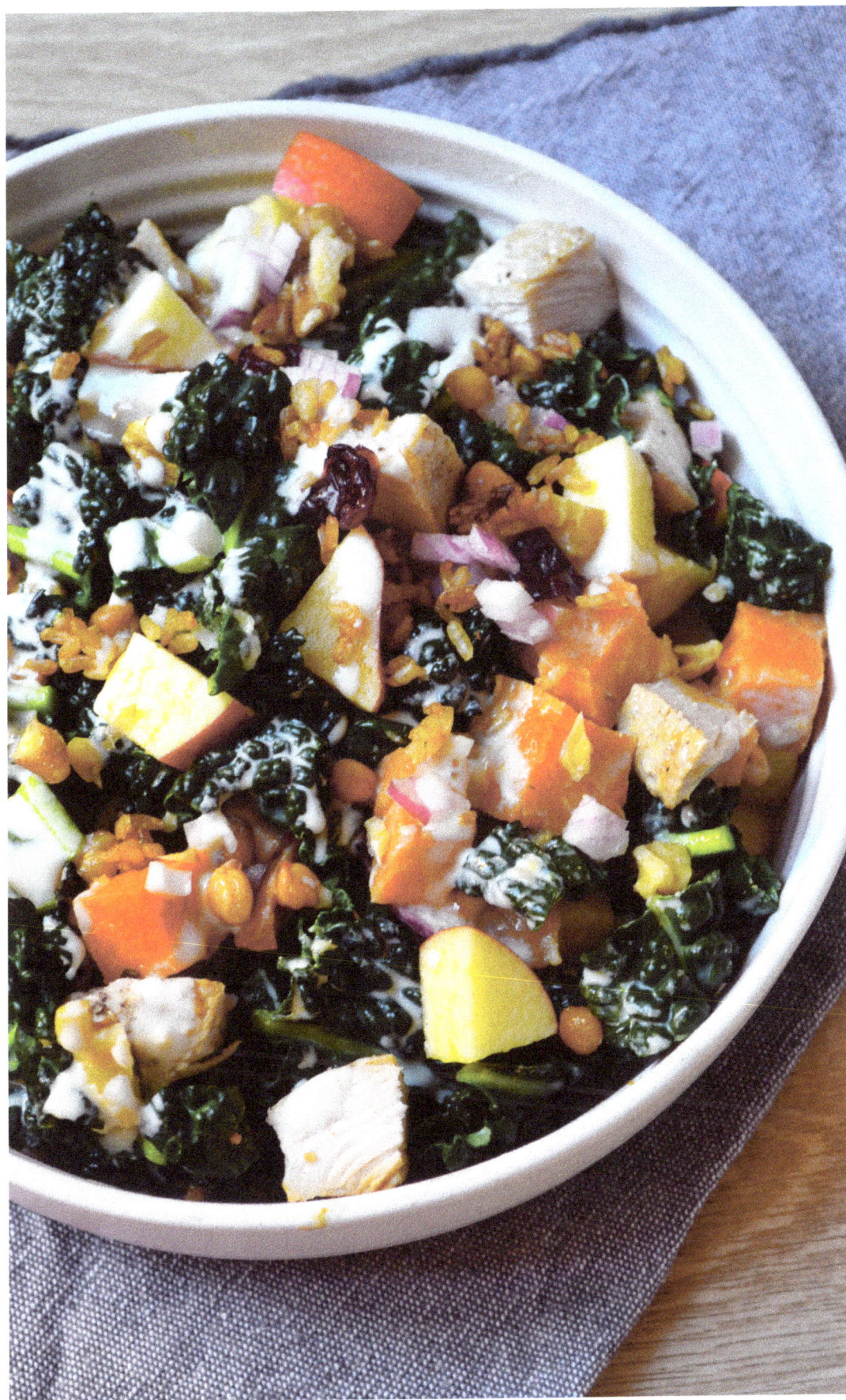

# ROOT VEGGIE SOUP

**Serves:** 4    **Prep:** 15 minutes    **Cook:** 45 minutes

1 tbsp olive oil
1 brown onion, chopped
750g kent pumpkin, peeled
  and chopped
2 carrots, peeled and
  chopped*
1 sweet potato, peeled and
  chopped*
1 apple, peeled and
  chopped*
2 tbsp thyme
¼ tsp cinnamon
¼ tsp nutmeg
4 cups vegetable stock (see
  page 243)
400g canned chickpeas,
  drained and rinsed
Pinch of salt and pepper

**Topping suggestions:**
Sunflower seeds, pepitas
  and olive oil
Roasted veggie peels and
  thyme sprigs (pictured)

Heat a large pot on medium and add olive oil. Add the onion and cook until softened.

Add the pumpkin, carrots and sweet potato, covering with a lid to soften, stirring every couple of minutes. Add the apple, thyme, cinnamon and nutmeg and stir.

Add the vegetable stock and bring to a boil. Reduce to simmer for about 25 minutes. Add the chickpeas and simmer for a further 5 minutes.

Once the vegetables have softened, remove from heat and use a stick blender to purée the vegetables. Season with salt and pepper.

Serve with toppings of choice.

**TIPS:**
› Place peels from the carrot, apple and potato onto a lined baking dish. Drizzle with olive oil and season with salt. Roast for 30 minutes until crispy. Use for serving.

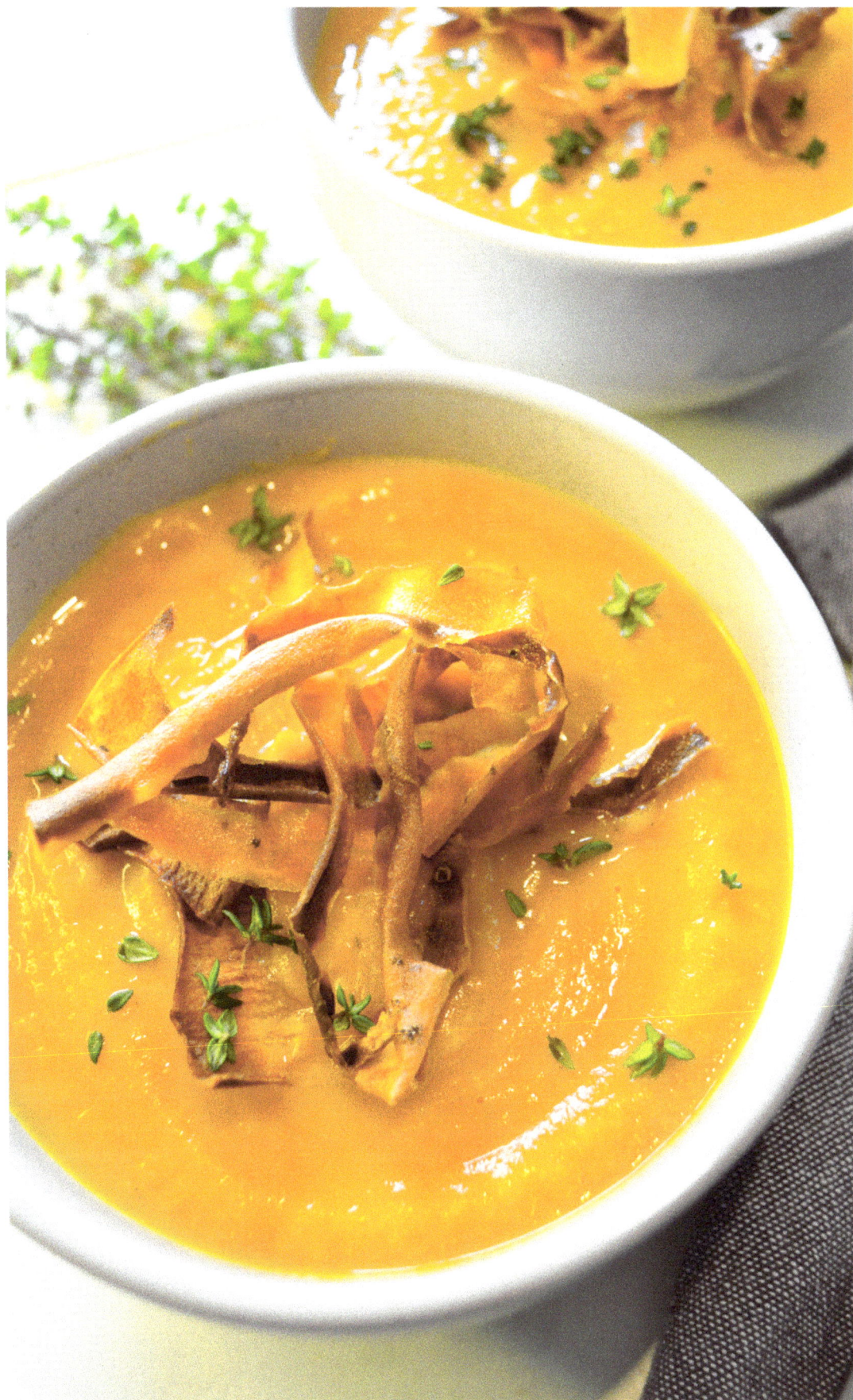

# TURKEY PATTIES
## WITH ROAST VEGGIES AND QUINOA

**Serves:** 4    **Prep:** 15 minutes    **Cook:** 50 minutes

**For the veggie medley:**
1 zucchini, sliced
1 carrot, sliced
½ butternut pumpkin, pealed and cubed
1 sweet potato, diced
1 red onion, sliced
¼ cauliflower, cut into florets
1 leek, sliced
Olive oil to drizzle
Balsamic vinegar to drizzle (optional)
Salt and pepper to taste
½ cup quinoa, cooked

**For the turkey patties:**
1 carrot, grated
1 zucchini, grated (squeezed out to remove excess water)
½ red chilli, diced
1 tbsp ground fennel seeds
500g turkey mince

**To serve:**
1 lemon, quartered (optional)

Preheat the oven to 200°C fan-forced.

On a lined baking tray, add all the chopped vegetables and drizzle with olive oil, balsamic vinegar and season with salt and pepper. Bake in the oven for 40 minutes.

In a bowl, add the grated carrot, zucchini, chilli, fennel seeds and turkey mince. Season with salt and pepper and stir to combine.

Take a heaped tablespoon scoop of turkey mince, roll into a ball and place on a plate. Repeat until all the mixture has been used. Set aside.

Cook the quinoa following the packet instructions.

When there is about 10-15 minutes left on the vegetables, heat a frypan on medium high with oil. Once heated, take a turkey mince ball, use your hands to flatten it into a patty and place in the frypan. Cook for 2-3 minutes and then flip. Cook for another 2-3 minutes, until cooked through.

Remove the vegetables from oven and stir them through the cooked quinoa. Serve on a plate and top with turkey patties.

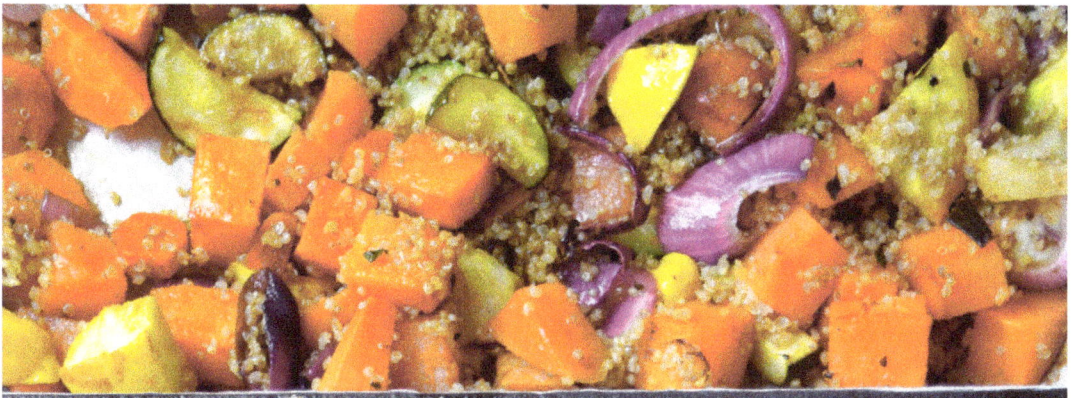

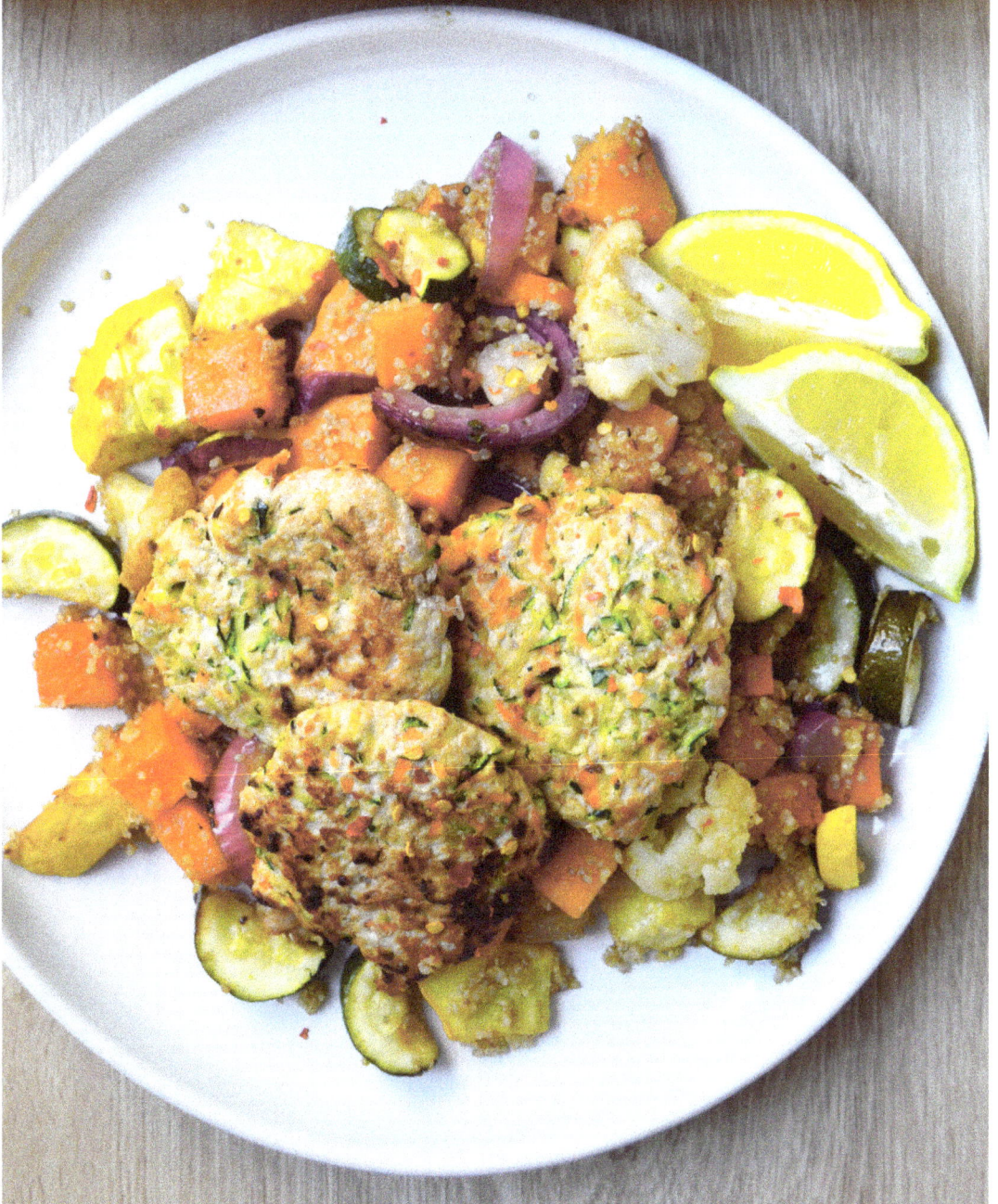

# CAULIFLOWER & LEEK SOUP

**Serves:** 4     **Prep:** 10 minutes     **Cook:** 30 minutes

1 tbsp olive oil
1 leek, sliced
2 garlic cloves
2 tbsp dried thyme
1 cauliflower, chopped (use
   leaves and core too)
800g canned white beans,
   drained and rinsed
4 cups vegetable stock (see
   page 243)
1 tbsp Dijon mustard
¼ cup parsley
Pinch of salt and pepper

**To serve:**
Almonds, roughly chopped
Parsley, chopped
Olive oil, to drizzle
Sprinkle of hemp seeds
Sourdough bread

Heat a large pot on medium and add olive oil. Add the leek and garlic and sauté for 3 minutes. Add the thyme and continue cooking for another 2 minutes.

Add the cauliflower, white beans and vegetable stock. Cover and bring to a boil before reducing to a simmer until the cauliflower is tender.

Add the Dijon, parsley, salt and pepper and stir through. Blend using a hand blender until smooth.

Top with almonds, more parsley and a drizzle of olive oil. Serve with sourdough bread.

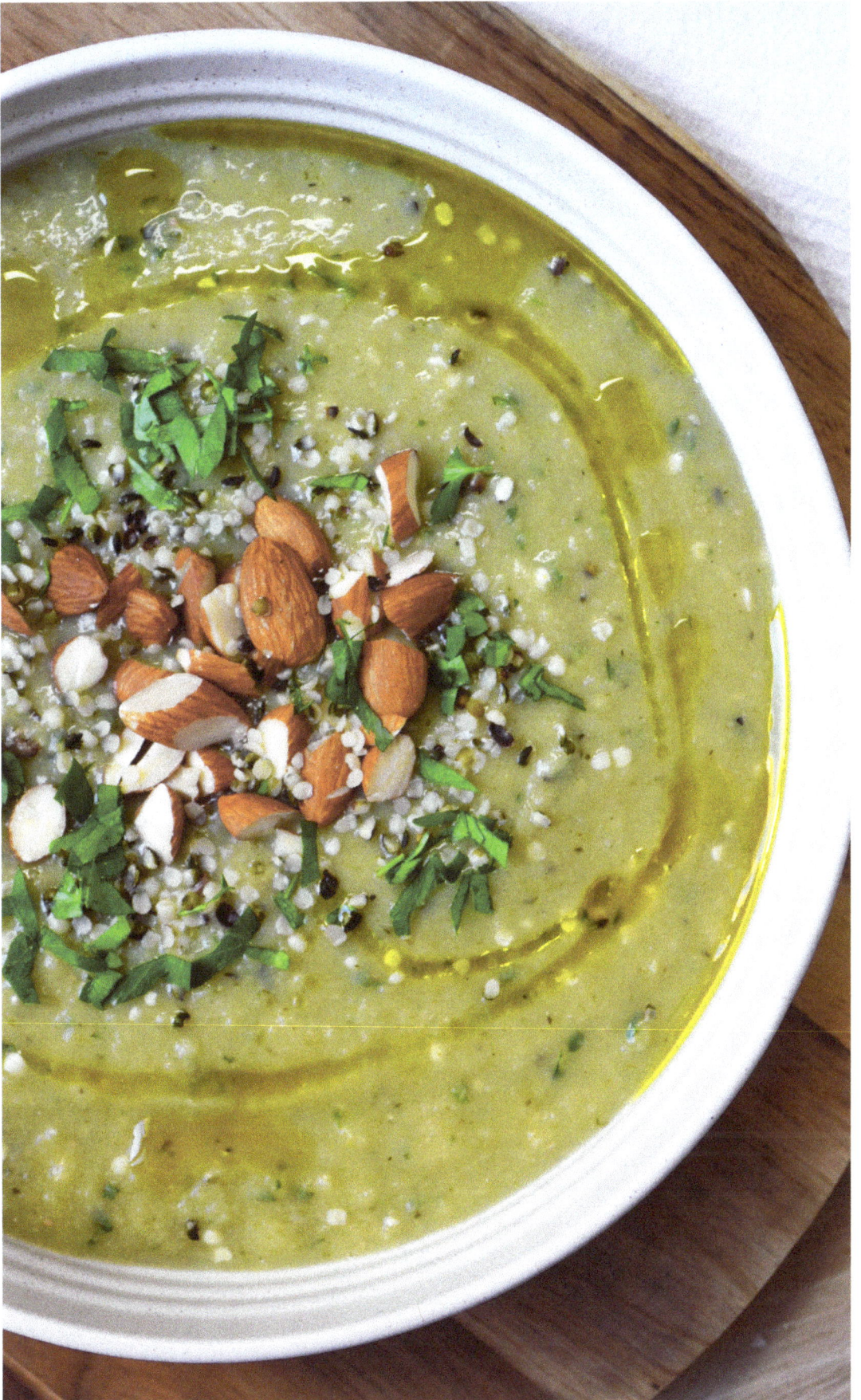

# DECONSTRUCTED SUSHI BOWLS

**Serves:** 4     **Prep:** 10 minutes     **Cook:** n/a

4 cans tuna, drained
2 cups brown rice, cooked
2 carrots, julienned
2 cucumbers, sliced
2 avocados, halved and
  sliced
Pickled ginger
Seaweed pieces/nori sheets
Sushi topping (see page 45)

**For the mayo:**
½ cup mayo of choice
Pinch of cayenne pepper
1 tbsp rice wine vinegar

Add the rice to the base of the bowl. Then top each bowl with a can of tuna, the vegetables, avocado, pickled ginger, nori and cucumber.

Drizzle with mayo and sprinkle with sushi toppings.

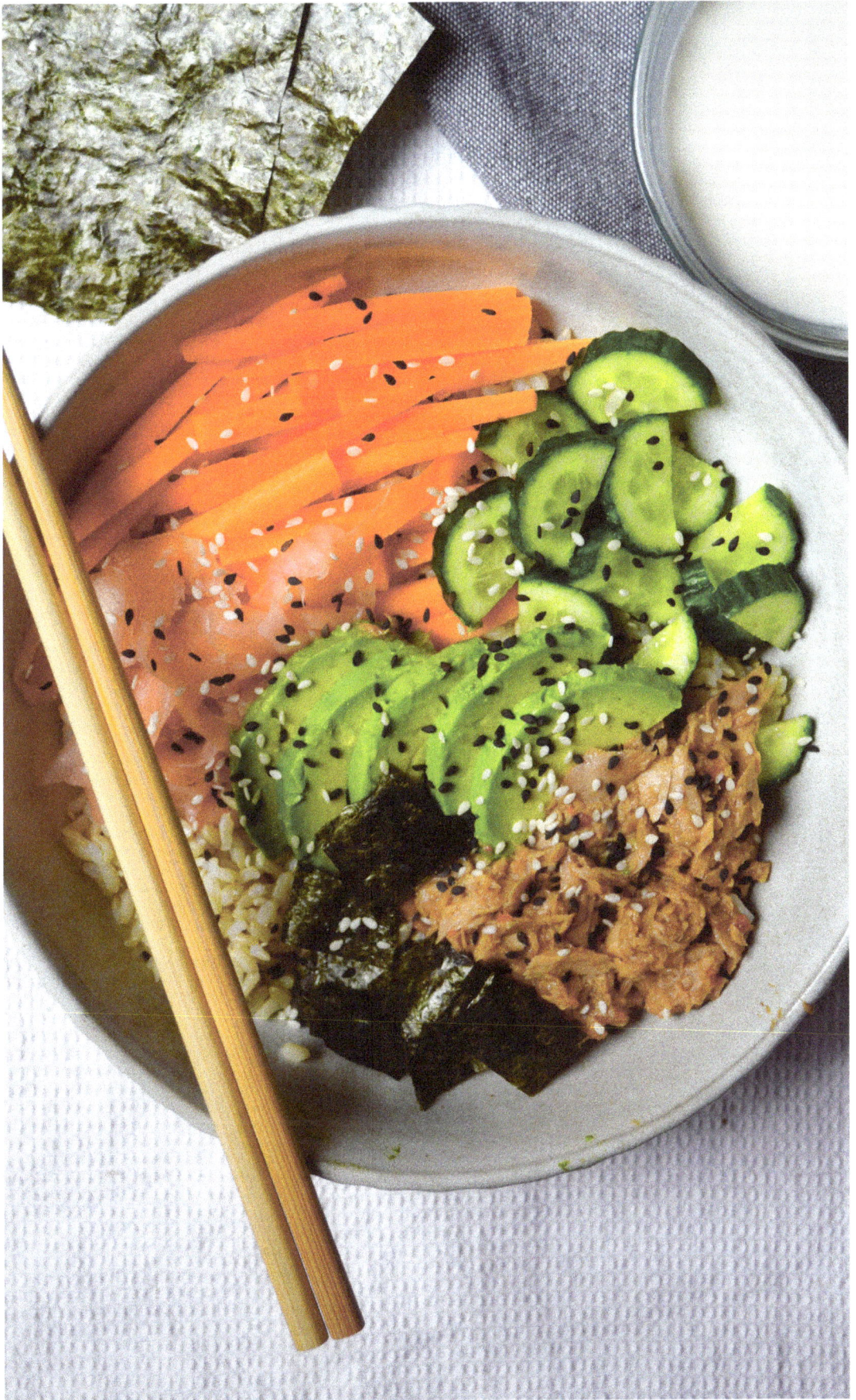

# CREAMY CHICKPEA & SWEET POTATO CURRY

**Serves:** 4     **Prep:** 15 minutes     **Cook:** 15 minutes

**For the curry:**
1 large sweet potato, diced
Olive oil
2 cloves garlic, minced
¼ bunch coriander, stalks
  finely chopped, leaves
  reserved for garnish
2 tbsp curry powder
  (adjusted to taste)
1 tbsp turmeric
2 tbsp tomato paste
800g canned cannellini
  beans, drained and rinsed
400ml coconut milk
4 tbsp nutritional yeast
8 tbsp sunflower seeds
2 tbsp almond butter
2 cup vegetable stock
800g canned chickpeas,
  drained and rinsed
4 cups baby spinach

**For the rice cabbage\*:**
1 small wombok cabbage,
  chopped into large chunks
2 garlic cloves
Olive oil
Pinch salt and pepper

Preheat the oven to 200°C fan-forced and line a baking tray.

Place the diced sweet potato on the baking tray and drizzle with olive oil. Bake in the oven for 25–30 minutes, until soft.

Meanwhile, add the garlic and coriander leaves to a heated pot with a little olive oil. Sauté for 2-3 minutes until softened. Add the curry powder, turmeric and tomato paste. Cook for a further 1 minute. Remove from heat and add to a blender, along with the cannellini beans, coconut milk, nutritional yeast, sunflower seeds, almond butter and vegetable stock.

Blend until a smooth and silky consistency has formed. Adjust the taste by adding more curry powder, if desired. Return to the pot and add in the cooked sweet potato, chickpeas and spinach. Cook on a medium heat, until the spinach has wilted and the sauce is warm.

Meanwhile, prepare the riced cabbage by adding the cabbage and garlic to a blender. Blend until a fine rice texture has formed. Add to a frypan with a small drizzle of olive oil and sauté for 4-5 minutes. Season with salt and pepper.

Once the rice is cooked, divide between the bowls and serve your curry over the top. Garnish with extra coriander leaves, if desired.

**NOTE**
› Alternatively, you can serve this with cauliflower rice or brown rice, as both are luteal phase hero ingredients

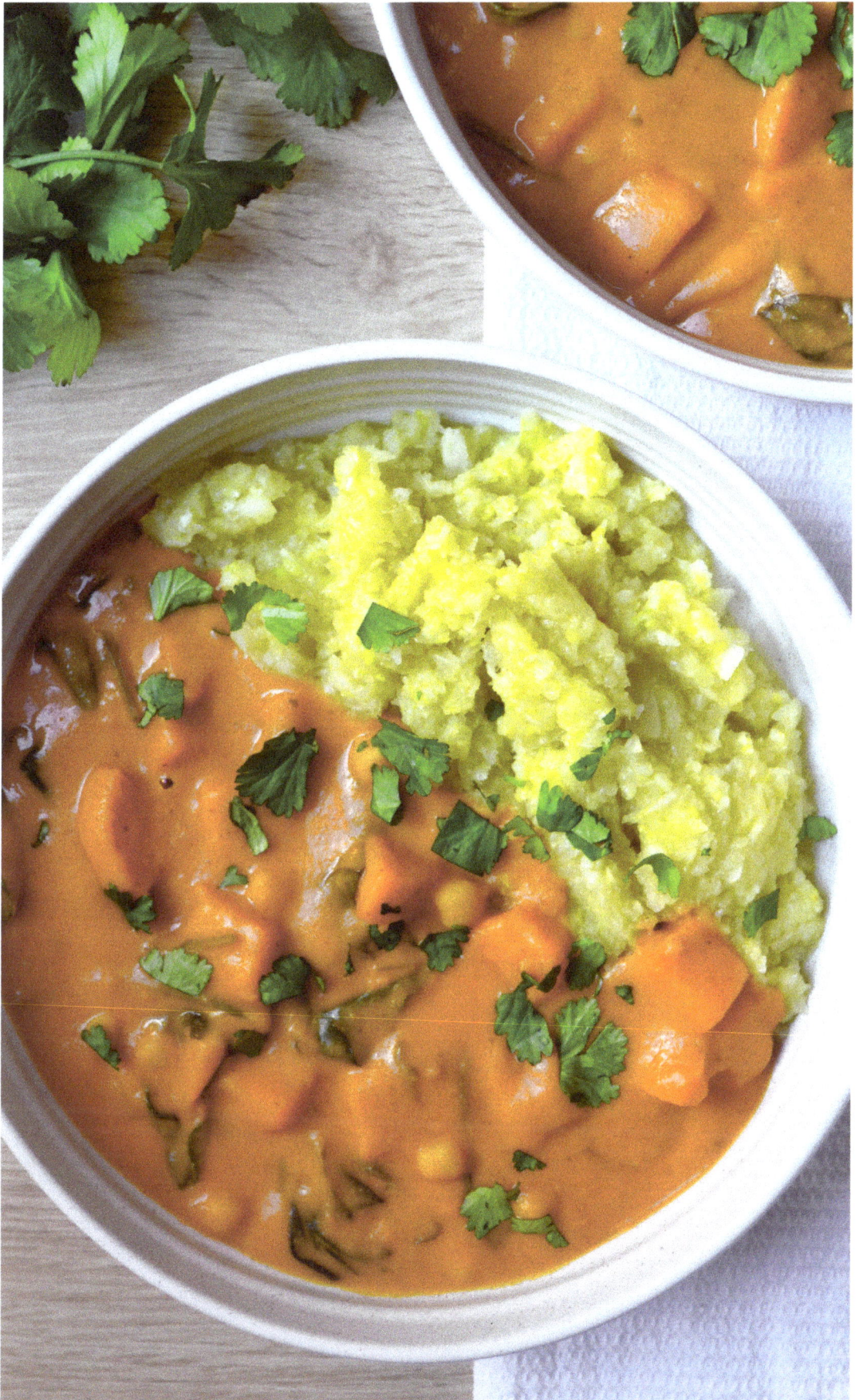

# TURKEY & ROASTED VEGGIE TRAY BAKE

**Serves:** 4     **Prep:** 15 minutes     **Cook:** 60 minutes

**For the turkey:**
4 turkey breasts
1 tbsp olive oil
1 tsp rosemary
1 tsp thyme
Pinch of salt and pepper

**For the veggies:**
1 large sweet potato, diced
2 carrots, chopped
1 fennel bulb, layers
  separated
¼ cup olive oil
1 tbsp rosemary
1 tbsp thyme
Pinch of salt and pepper
1 large red onion, thinly
  sliced
2 granny smith apples,
  sliced
1 tbsp apple cider vinegar

Preheat the oven to 200°C fan-forced.

In a bowl, add the turkey breast, olive oil, rosemary, thyme and salt and pepper. Stir to combine until well coated. Stand aside.

Add the sweet potato, carrots and fennel to a baking dish. Drizzle with olive oil, and top with rosemary, thyme, salt and pepper. Bake in the oven for 35 minutes.

Add the onions, apples and apple cider vinegar to the baking tray and bake for another 10 minutes.

Add the turkey breasts to the baking tray, laying them on top of the vegetables. Bake for 10 minutes.

Once cooked, remove from the oven and serve.

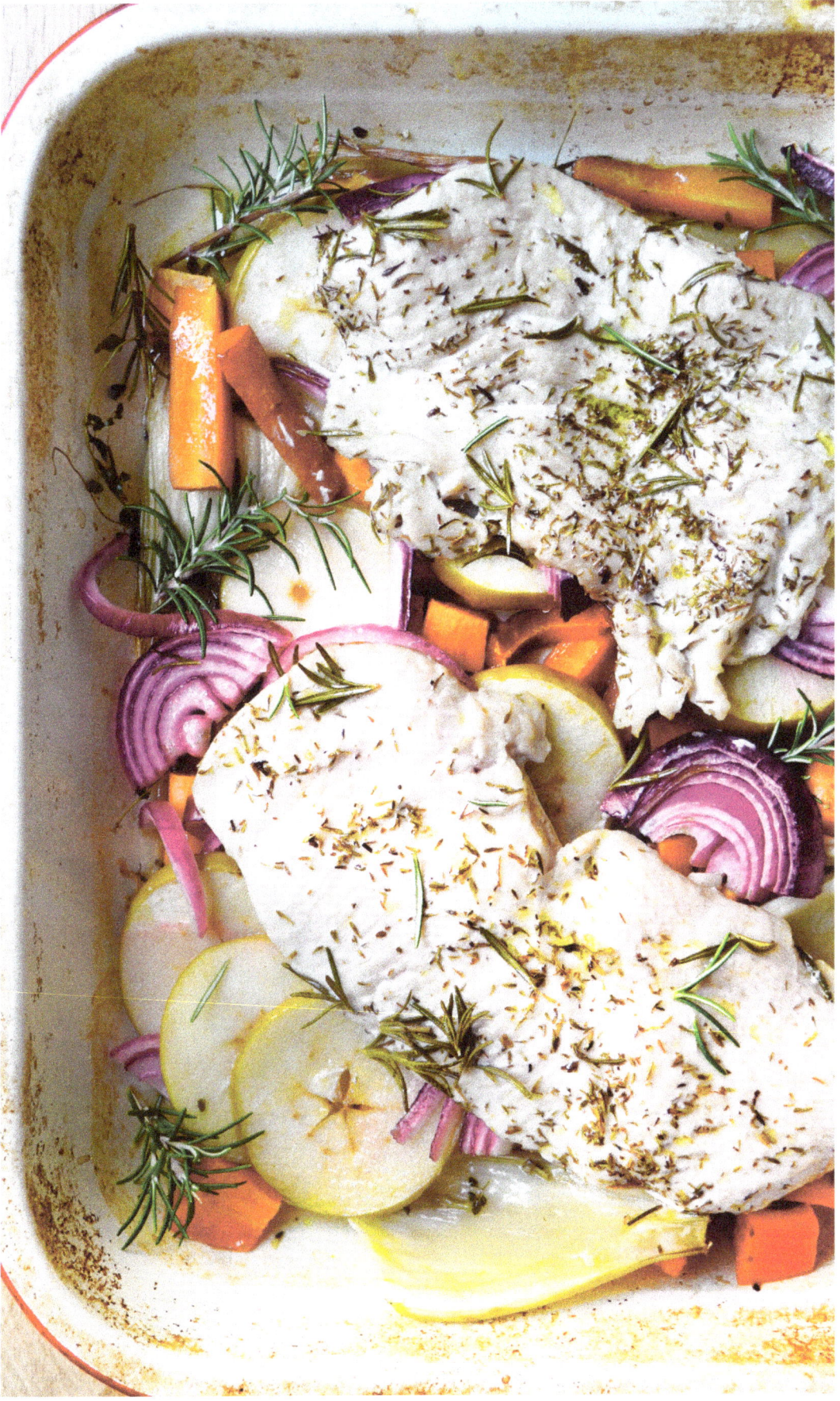

# snacks

Baked Apples &
Walnut Crumble

Hummus Dip

Roasted Chickpeas
Two Ways

Apple Crumble
Bliss Balls

Millet &
Seed Bars

Chocolate Coated
Nutty Dates

# BAKED APPLES & WALNUT CRUMBLE

**Serves:** 4      **Prep:** 5 minutes      **Cook:** 30 minutes

4 apples, peeled and
  chopped
1 tbsp water
1 tsp cinnamon
¼ cup walnuts
¼ cup oats
¼ cup sunflower seeds
1 tbsp maple syrup

**To serve:**
Greek yoghurt (1 cup per
  serve)
Fresh fruit
Honey/maple syrup

Preheat the oven to 180°C fan-forced.

Add the apples into a saucepan on medium heat with the water and cinnamon. Cover the saucepan with a lid and allow apples to cook for 10 minutes or until tender.

Meanwhile in a food processor, add the walnuts, oats, sunflower seeds and maple syrup. Blitz until ingredients are combined.

Once the apples are cooked, place them in a baking dish and top with the walnut crumb.

Bake in the oven for about 20 minutes or until the crumb is lightly golden.

Serve with yoghurt, fresh fruit and a drizzle of honey or maple syrup.

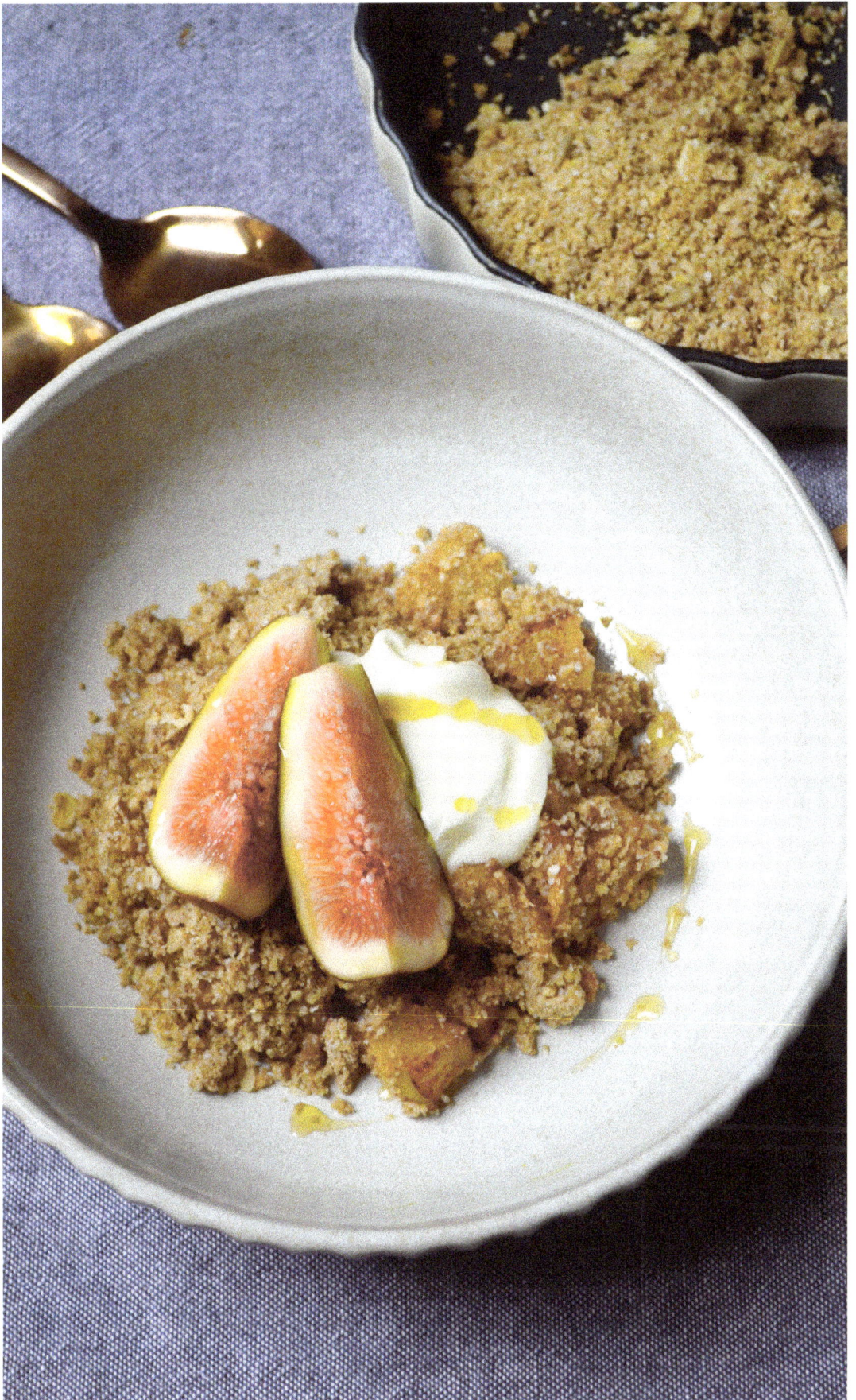

# HUMMUS DIP

**Serves:** 1    **Prep:** 5 minutes    **Cook:** n/a

**For the dip:**
400g canned chickpeas,
  drained and rinsed
1 garlic clove
½ tbsp ground cumin
1 lemon, juiced
3 tbsp tahini
3 tbsp olive oil
¼ cup warm water

**For the topping (optional):**
Roasted chickpeas
  (see page 233)
Pinch of sweet paprika
Drizzle of olive oil
Pine nuts

**To serve:**
Vegetable sticks
Linseed crackers
  (see page 251)

In a food processor, add all the dip ingredients except the water and blend until smooth. Then add the water and continue to blend until smooth.

Transfer to a bowl and serve with a drizzle of olive oil and sprinkle with paprika if desired.

Serve with vegetable sticks and/or seed crackers.

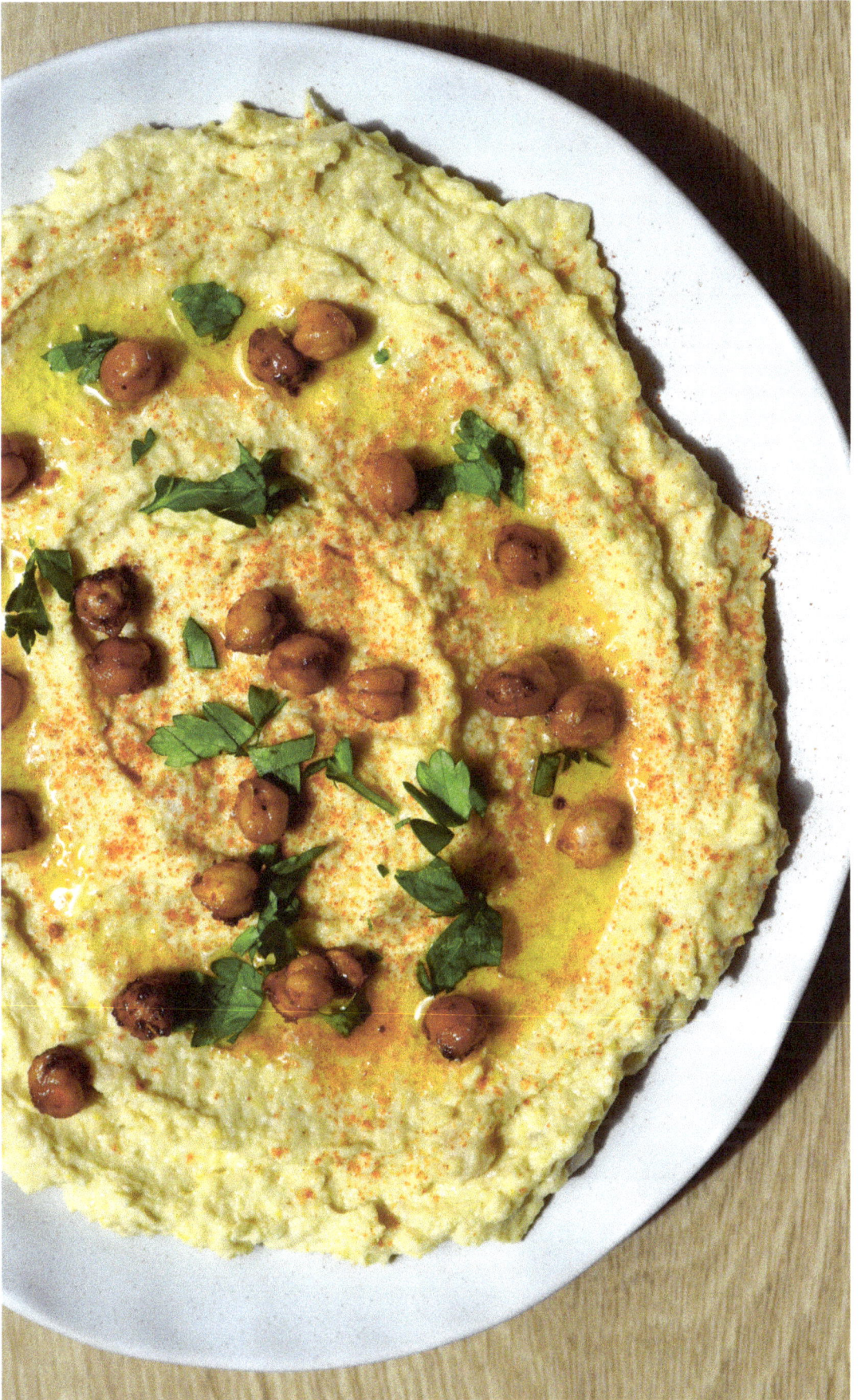

# ROASTED CHICKPEAS TWO WAYS

**Serves:** 1     **Prep:** 5 minutes     **Cook:** 50-60 minutes

400g canned chickpeas,
  drained and rinsed

Savoury:
1 tsp ground cumin
½ tsp garlic powder
½ tsp dried thyme
Pinch of salt and pepper
1 tbsp olive oil

Sweet:
1 tbsp coconut oil, melted
1 tsp cacao powder
½ tsp cinnamon
1 tsp maple syrup
2 squares of dark chocolate,
  melted

Preheat the oven to 200°C fan-forced.

Toss the chickpeas with the chosen flavour ingredients (sweet or savoury) and then add to a lined baking tray.

Roast in the oven until dry and crispy: 50 minutes for the savoury chickpeas and 60 minutes for the sweet chickpeas.

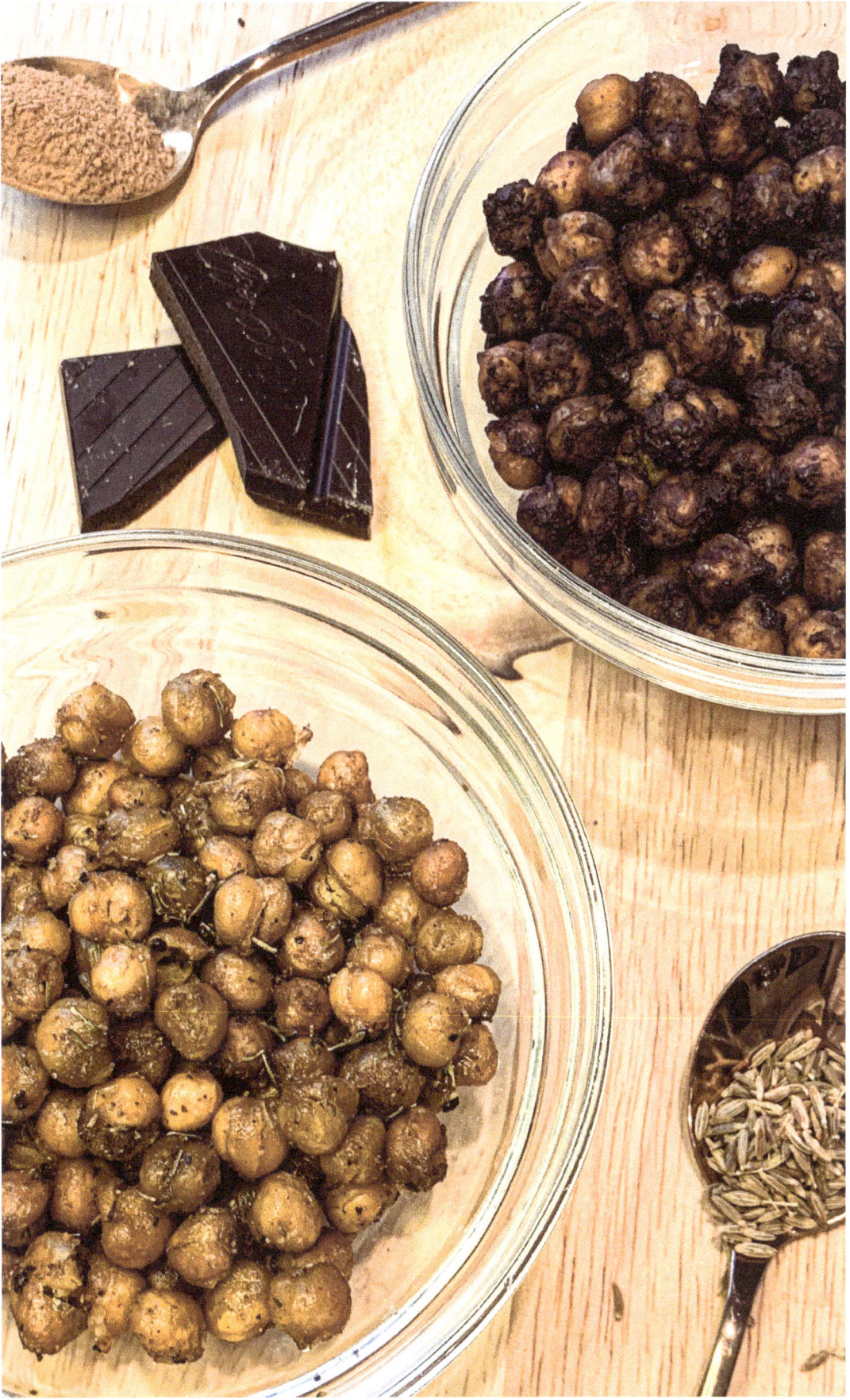

# APPLE CRUMBLE BLISS BALLS

**Serves:** 8-10 balls     **Prep:** 5 minutes     **Cook:** 30 minutes

2 apples
¼ cup desiccated coconut
  (plus extra for coating)
4 medjool dates, pitted
½ cup rolled oats
½ tsp cinnamon
1 scoop vanilla protein
  powder

Grate the apples with skin on into a bowl and squeeze out excess moisture.

In a food processor, add the coconut, dates, oats and cinnamon. Blend until a fine mixture forms.

Add the oat mixture to the apples and mix to combine. In tablespoon heaps, roll out the mixture into balls. Coat the balls in the dessicated coconut.

Place on a plate or tray and refrigerate to set.

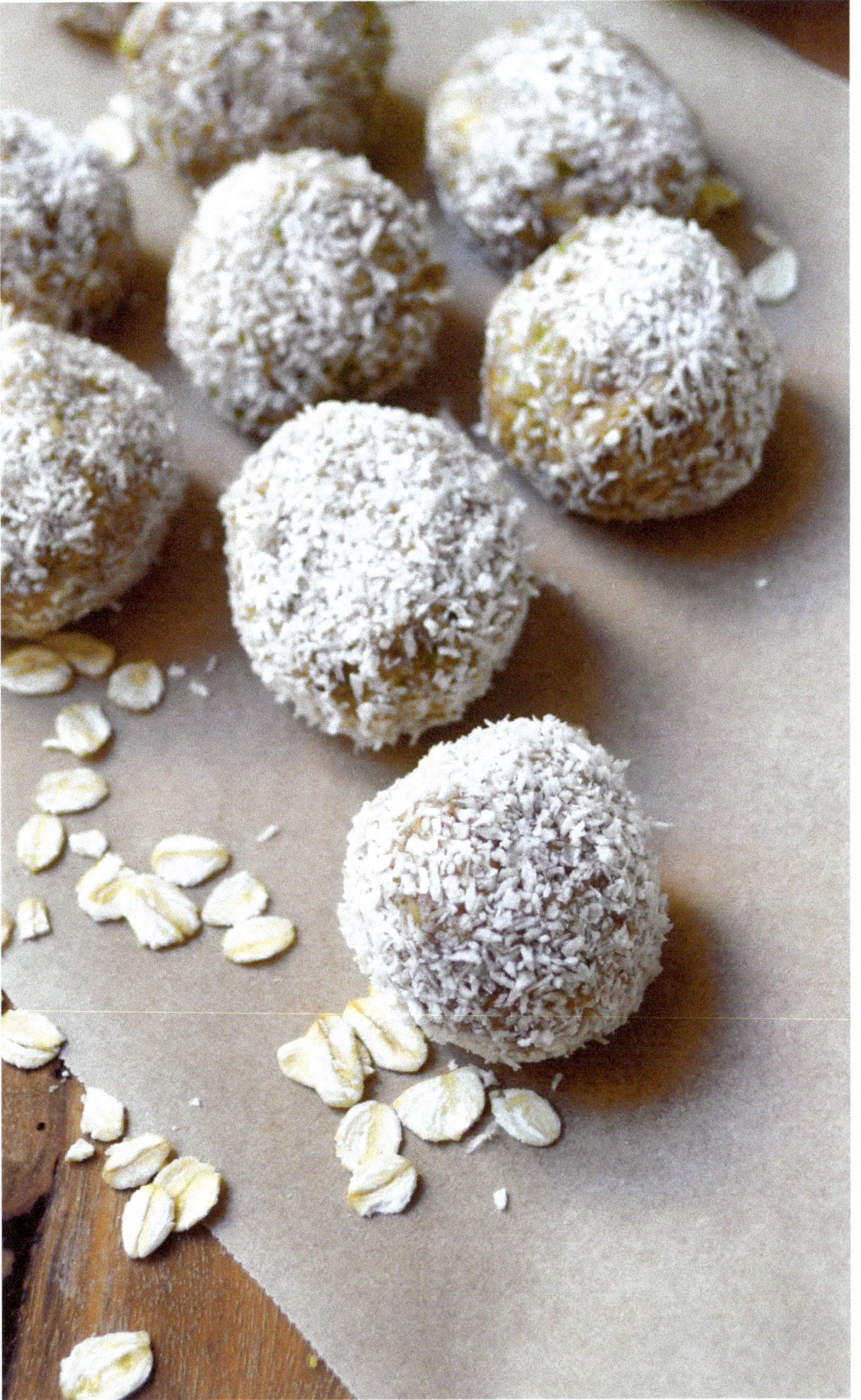

# MILLET & SEED BARS

**Serves:** 8 bars     **Prep:** 5 minutes     **Cook:** 50 minutes

**For the bars:**
1 banana
8 medjool dates
½ cup rolled oats
1 cup millet
¼ cup pepita seeds
¼ cup sunflower seeds
¼ cup desiccated coconut
¼ cup flaxseed
1 tbsp coconut oil, melted

**For the chocolate drizzle:**
**(Optional)**
1 tbsp coconut oil
1 tbsp cacao

Preheat the oven to 180°C fan-forced.

Add all the ingredients into a food processor and blend to combine. Transfer the mixture into a lined 20x20 oven dish and press down to create an even layer.

Bake in the oven for approximately 40 minutes or until the top starts to turn golden and the middle is semi-firm.

Remove from the oven and allow to cool. Slice into bars.

For the chocolate drizzle, add the coconut oil and the cacao in a small bowl. Mix to combine well. Drizzle immediately over the bars.

Store in an airtight container.

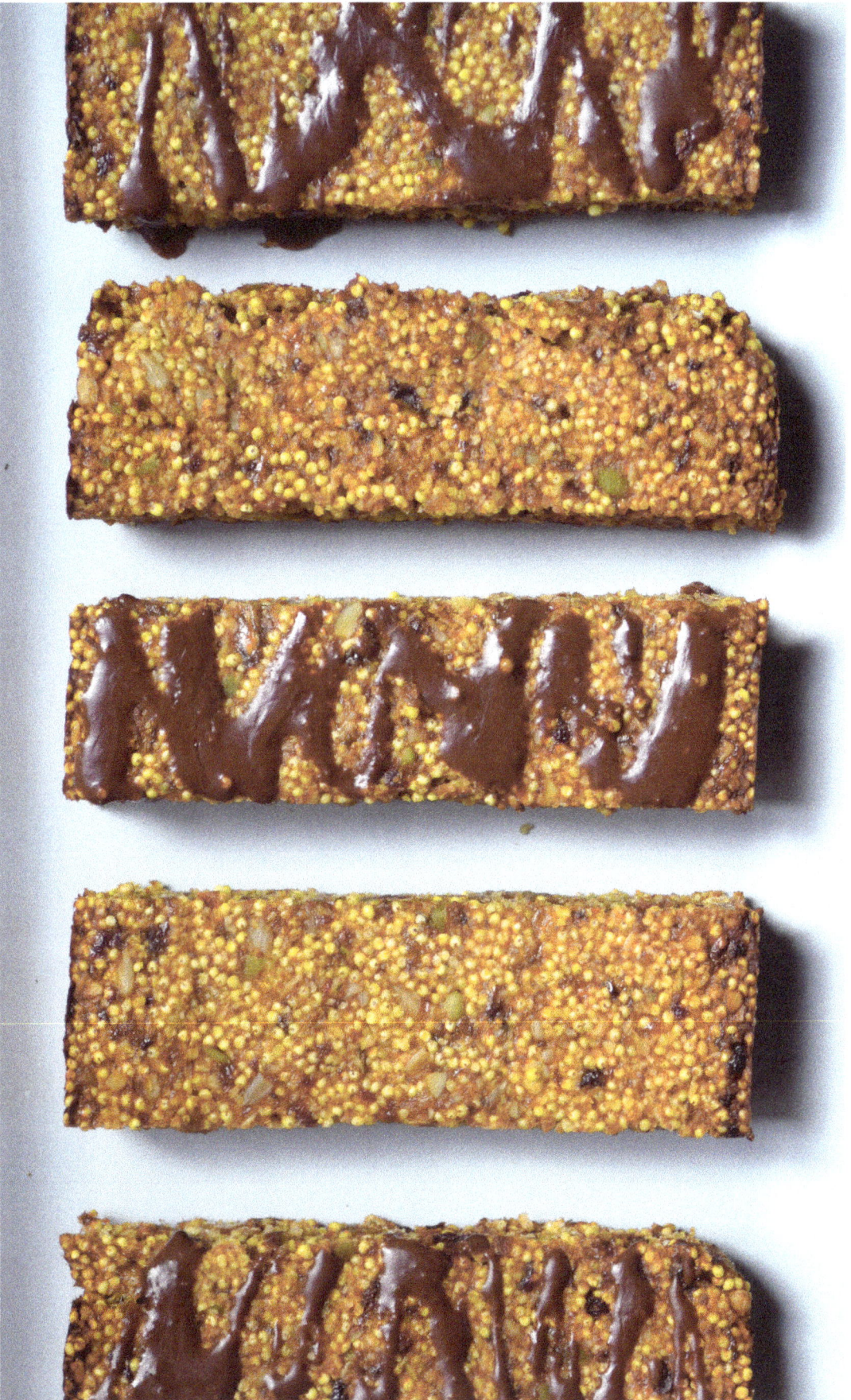

# CHOCOLATE COATED NUTTY DATES

**Serves:** 10     **Prep:** 15 minutes     **Cook:** 10 minutes

10 medjool dates
1 tbsp nut butter of choice
¼ cup cacao powder
¼ cup coconut oil, melted
1 tsp flaxseed meal
¼ tsp cinnamon

Topping suggestions:
1 tbsp chia seeds
1 tbsp pumpkin seeds/
   sunflower seeds/goji
   berries (chopped)
1 tbsp crushed nuts

Slice through the top of the dates to remove the seeds, while also ensuring the date remains whole.

Use a knife to fill the centre of the dates with nut butter before closing the edges together and placing on a plate. Refrigerate while making the chocolate coating.

To make the melted chocolate, combine the cacao powder and coconut oil in a small bowl, stirring until the cacao is smooth. Stir in the flaxseed meal and cinnamon.

Roll the dates in the chocolate to coat them evenly and refrigerate for 5 minutes. After that layer has set, double dip the dates in the remaining chocolate and sprinkle with crushed nuts, chopped seeds/goji berries immediately.

Refrigerate until set.

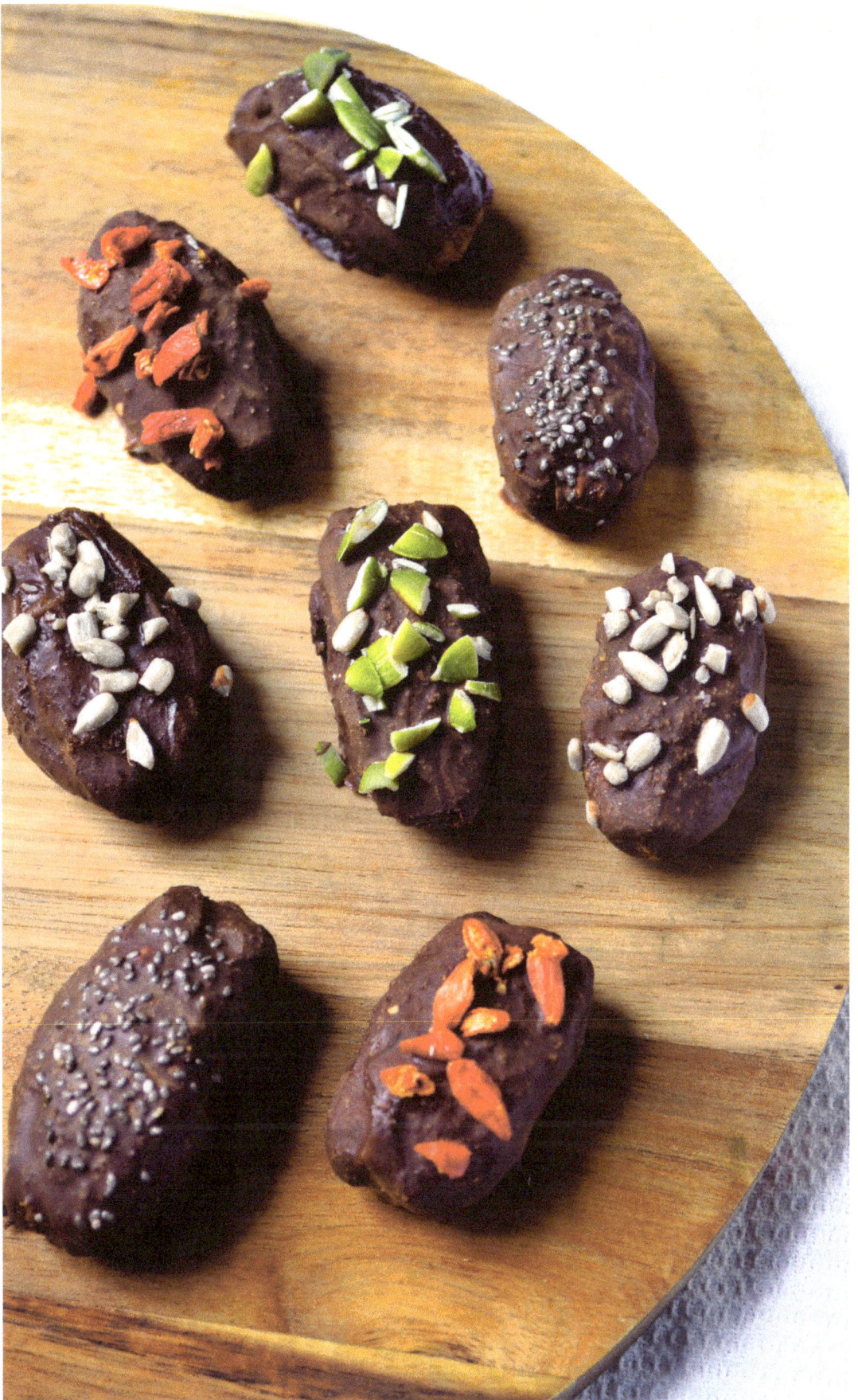

nourishing
basics

# basics

Homemade
Veggie Stock

Homemade
Bone Broth

Adrenal Cocktail

Pickled Vegetables

Balsamic Vinegar &
Caramelised Onion
Linseed Crackers

Immunity Booster

Grain Free
Granola

# HOMEMADE VEGGIE STOCK

**Serves:** 1    **Prep:** 5 minutes    **Cook:** 60 minutes

1 onion, chopped
1 carrot, chopped
Vegetable scraps, fresh
  or frozen (e.g., broccoli
  stems, herb stems, peels,
  leek tops, potato ends)
Dried herbs (e.g., thyme,
  oregano, basil)
Fresh herbs (rosemary)
1.5L water (filtered, if
  possible)
Olive oil
1 tbsp salt
1 tbsp pepper

In a large pot heated to medium with olive oil, add the onion and carrot and sauté for 5 minutes. Add the vegetable scraps and herbs of choice and cook for a further 5 minutes.

Add the water and bring to a boil. Reduce to a simmer for 45 minutes. Season with salt and pepper.

Using a sieve, strain the liquid into a separate bowl. Use immediately or let it cool and store in a jar/container in the fridge or freezer.

**NOTE:**
› You can use store bought as well if short on time, but homemade will be more flavourful and have less preservatives and additives.

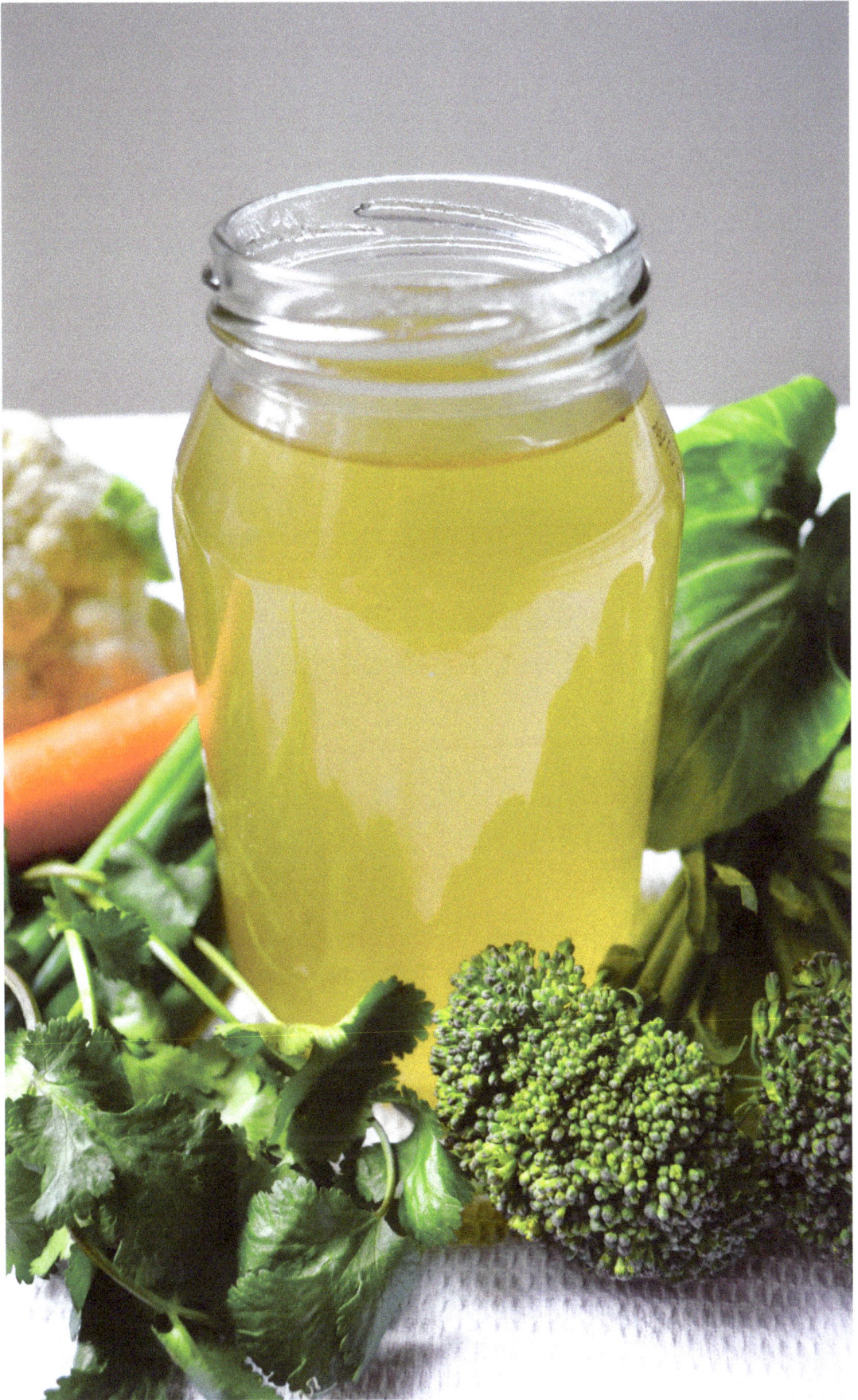

# HOMEMADE BONE BROTH

**Serves:** 1    **Prep:** 5 minutes    **Cook:** 3 hours

1 kg beef or lamb marrow
  bones (or the left over
  bones of a roast)
1 carrot, chopped
1 onion, chopped
2 garlic cloves
Vegetable scraps
2 tbsp herbs of choice
  (thyme, oregano,
  rosemary)
1 tbsp salt
1 tsp pepper
5-8 litres of water

Preheat the oven to 220°C fan-forced.

In a large pot on medium high heat, add the marrow bones and cover with water. Boil for 5 minutes, then drain and discard the water. Rinse the bones. This step will remove impurities and coagulated protein). Clean out the pot.

Add the marrow bones and the vegetable scraps to a tray and roast in the oven for 45 minutes. (This step enhances the flavour, but can be omitted if short on time).

In a large pot with the water, add all the ingredients and bring to a boil. Then reduce to a simmer for 1.5-2 hours. Remove from heat and allow to stand for 20 minutes.

Place a sieve over a bowl and drain the broth from the ingredients.

Store in sterilised glass jars or containers for 3 days or store in the freezer for 3 months. Enjoy in soups, stews or on its own. To serve on its own, simple reheat in a pot on the stove.

**NOTE:**
› If using leftover bones that have already been cooked (roast chicken, roast lamb bone), skip step 1-3 and go straight to adding all ingredients to the pot. You'll also require 3 litres less water by skipping step 2.

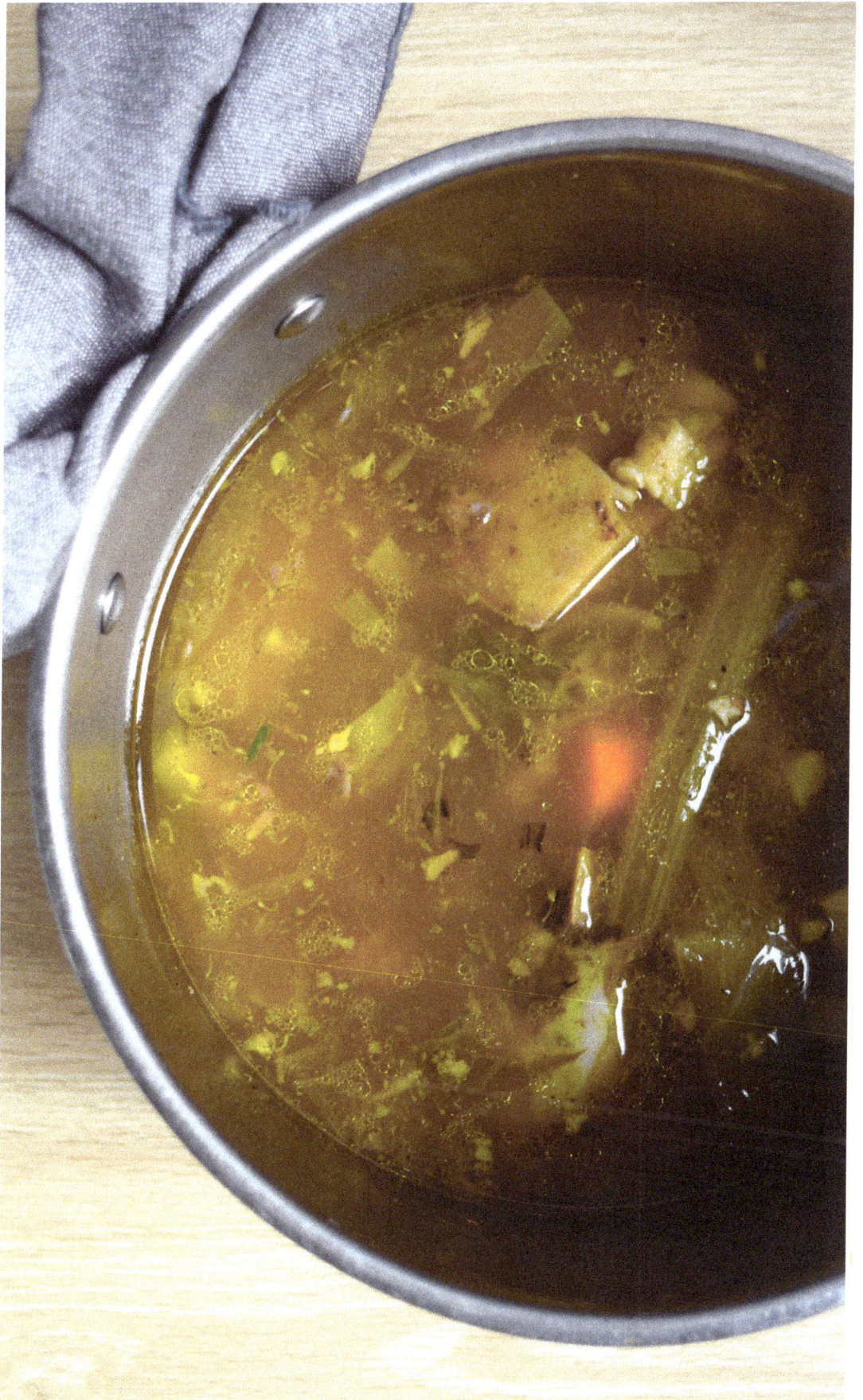

# ADRENAL COCKTAIL

Our adrenals become overworked and slow down when we experience too much stress. When this happens, it can also impact our body's ability to absorb nutrients, which we need to support our adrenals. This adrenal 'cocktail' contains simple ingredients that are rich in key nutrients like magnesium, vitamin C, potassium, sodium, calcium and phosphorus.

**Serves:** 1    **Prep:** 5 minutes    **Cook:** N/A

⅓ cup coconut water
⅓ cup mineral water
⅓ cup orange juice
1 heaped tablespoon
  magnesium powder
Pinch of celtic sea salt

Combine all the ingredients into a cup and stir.

Serve immediately or store in the refrigerator for up to 4 days in a bottle or jar.

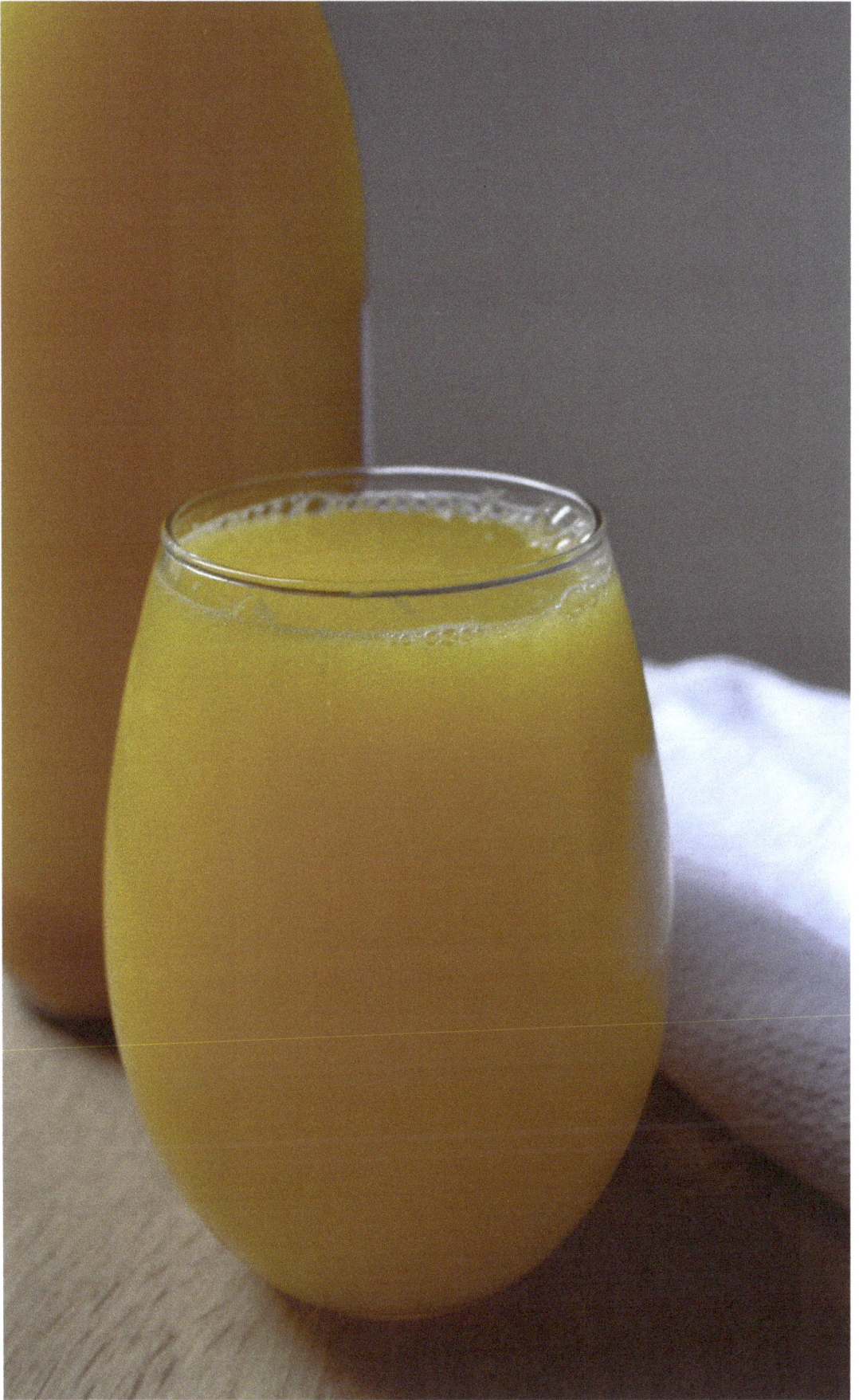

# PICKLED VEGETABLES

**Serves:** 1     **Prep:** 5 minutes     **Cook:** Overnight

**For the pickle base:**
½ cup white vinegar*
½ cup water*
1 tsp sugar

**Vegetable options:**
Red onion/white onion,
  thinly sliced
Carrot, grated or julienned
Cucumber, sliced (pictured)
  with dill and mustard
  seeds

In a small bowl, add all the ingredients for the pickle base and stir to combine.

Choose your preferred vegetables for pickling, such as thinly sliced red or white onion, grated or julienned carrot and sliced cucumber with dill and mustard seeds.

Place the prepared vegetables in a sterilised jar and pour the pickle base over the vegetables, ensuring they are fully submerged.

Seal the jar and store it in the refrigerator. Allow to pickle overnight.

**NOTE:**
› The amount will vary based on the size of the jars being used. You just need an equal amount of both.

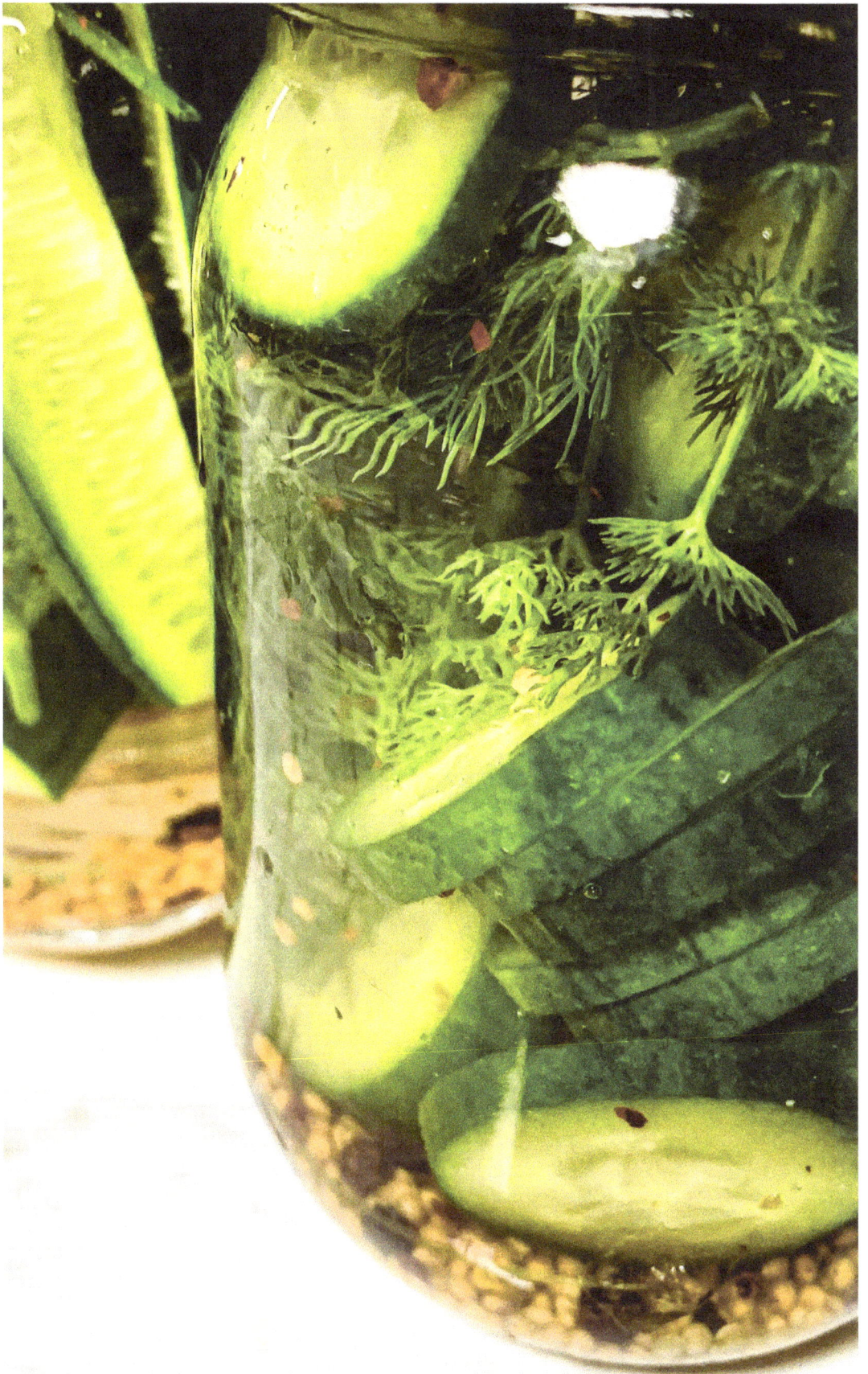

# BALSAMIC VINEGAR & CARAMELISED ONION LINSEED CRACKERS

**Serves:** 8 bars      **Prep:** 5 minutes      **Cook:** 60 minutes

½ cup linseeds
¼ cup pepitas
¼ cup sunflower seeds
1 tbsp sesame seeds
3 tbsp flaxseed meal
3 tbsp almond meal
2 tsp garlic powder
3 tbsp onion flakes/powder
3 tbsp balsamic vinegar
¾ cup water

Preheat the oven to 180°C fan-forced.

Combine all the ingredients in a bowl and allow to stand for 15 minutes or until the mixture is thick.

On a lined baking tray, press the mixture down until a thin, even layer has formed.

Bake in the oven for 30 minutes. Remove from the oven and allow to cool for 10 minutes.

Cut into cracker-shaped pieces or bars.

Reduce the oven temperature to 150°C fan-forced and return the crackers to the oven for a further 10 minutes to crisp.

Allow to cool before eating.

Store in an airtight container.

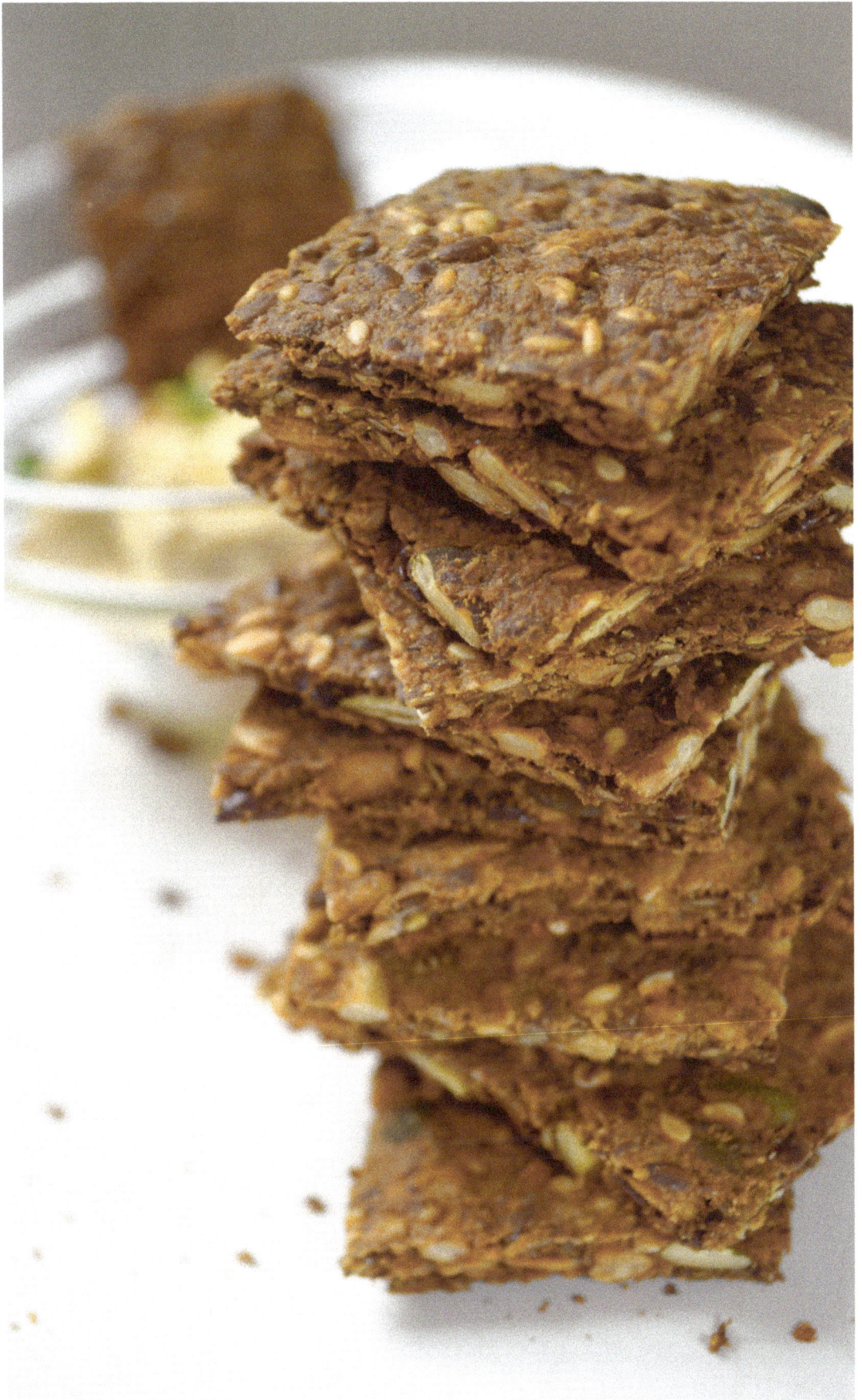

# IMMUNITY BOOSTER

Rich in zinc and magnesium, this immunity booster supports overall health, while copper aids in forming red blood cells and fighting infections. Particularly beneficial during pregnancy, the luteal phase and menstruation, this drink helps bolster the immune system when it's more vulnerable. Consuming it regularly can speed up recovery from illnesses and help fend off infections.

**Serves:** 1     **Prep:** 5 minutes     **Cook:** N/A

3-4 oranges, peeled
1 lemon, peeled
1 tbsp apple cider vinegar
1 cup water
1 thumb size piece of ginger
1 garlic clove, peeled
1 tbsp turmeric
1 tbsp manuka honey
Pinch of cayenne pepper
Pinch of black pepper

Blend all the ingredients together in a food processor.

Pour through a sieve or use a cheesecloth bag to separate the pulp from the juice.

Store in glass bottles and drink for the duration of an illness or use as a preventative measure.

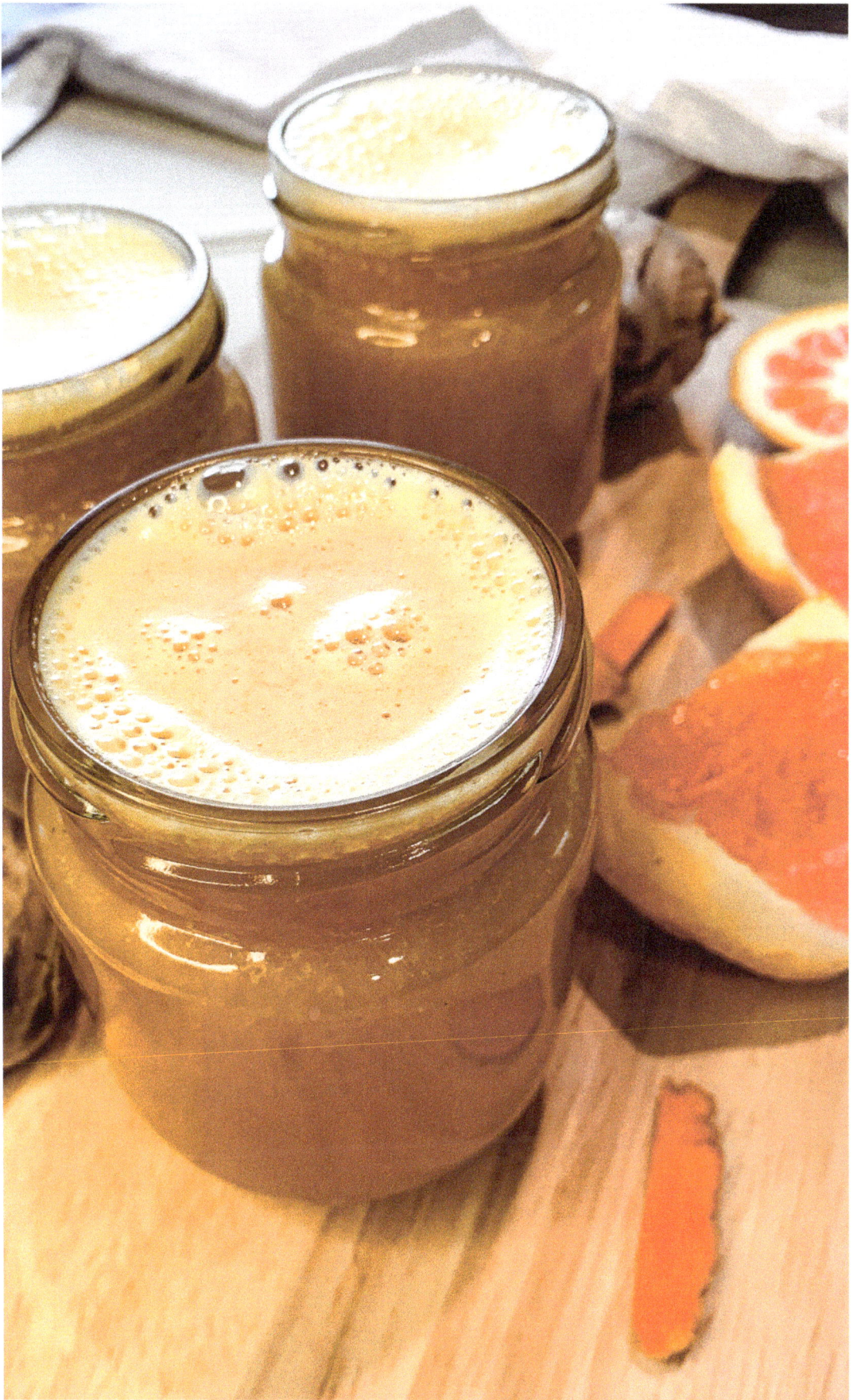

# GRAIN FREE GRANOLA

**Serves:** 1   **Prep:** 5 minutes   **Cook:** 30-40 minutes

½ cup almonds, roughly chopped
½ cup cashews, roughly chopped
½ cup walnuts, roughly chopped
¼ cup pepitas
¼ cup sunflower seeds
¼ cup coconut flakes
1 tbsp flaxseed meal
1 tbsp chia seeds
2 tbsp dried cranberries, chopped
1 tsp cinnamon
1 tbsp maple syrup
¼ cup coconut oil, melted

Preheat the oven to 180°C fan-forced.

Combine all the ingredients in a bowl and then transfer to a lined baking tray.

Bake in the oven for 30-40 minutes or until the nuts and seeds are roasted to your preference.

Allow to cool and store in an airtight container. Use in multiple recipes throughout this book.

**MAKE IT A TRAIL MIX:**
To turn this into a trail mix for on-the-go enjoyment, keep the nuts whole and add some dark chocolate pieces after baking for an extra treat.

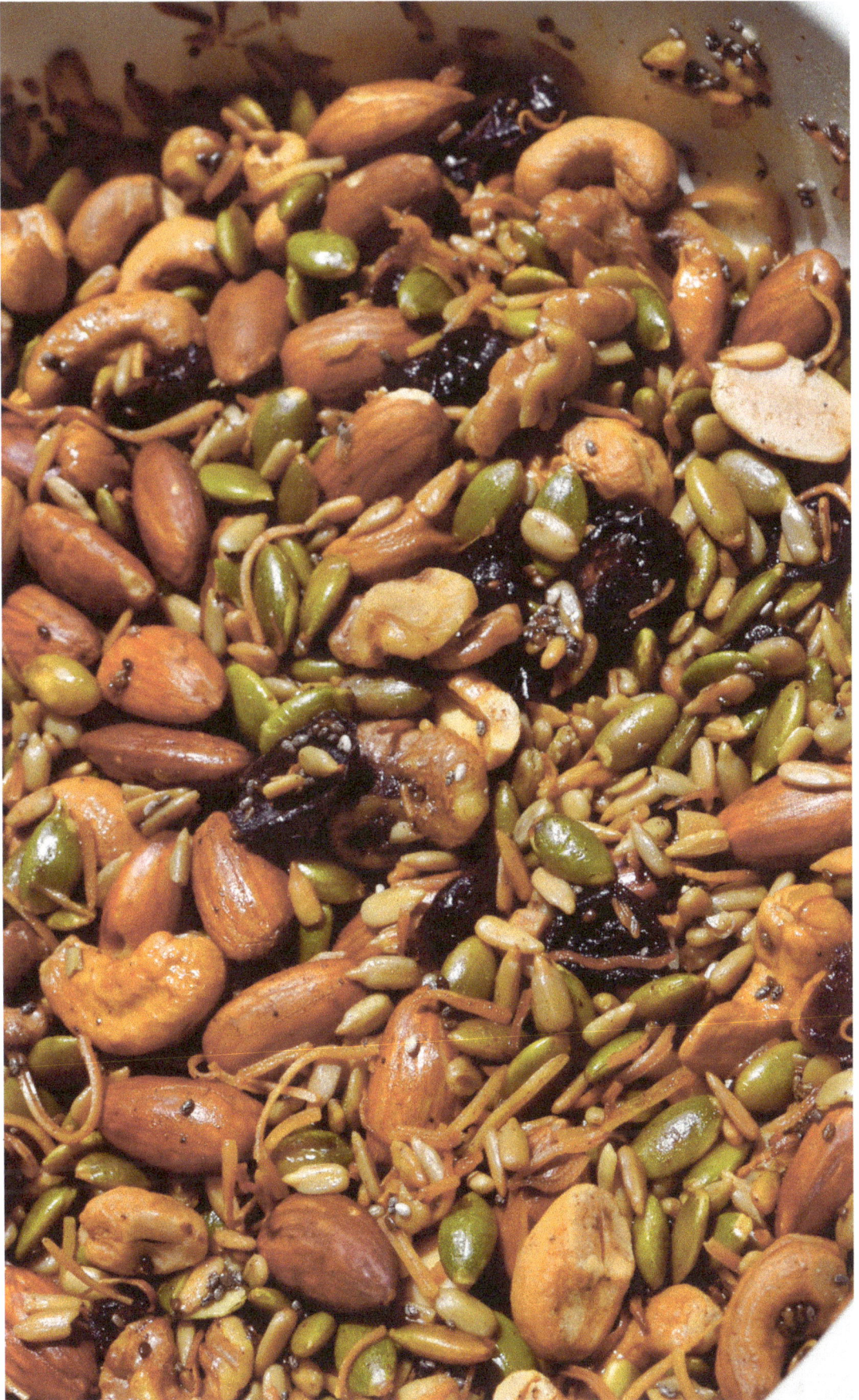

# ACKNOWLEDGEMENTS

I would like to thank my phenomenal family and friends who have supported me so wholeheartedly on this journey. From the very beginning, you were curious about what I was cooking and which phase of the cycle each meal was for. You were the ones who planted the seed that I could one day write a cookbook.

To my incredible friend Pamela – I am beyond grateful for you. You've been by my side from the very beginning when this idea was called *Moon Menu* then *Food for Your Flow* and finally *Nourish to Flourish*. You saw every stage of this evolution and used your incredible design skills to bring my vision to life. I'll never forget sitting in my living room together, dreaming and holding the vision of one day walking into a bookstore and seeing our creation on the shelf. The dream is now a reality and I couldn't have done it without you. Every woman needs a friend who can see her vision and help her create it. You are the best.

To my mum and dad, and my extended family, thank you for always supporting my dreams, encouraging me through moments of doubt and tough decisions, for sampling my food and giving honest feedback, and for listening (patiently!) as I talked endlessly about menstrual cycles, hormones and my next big idea.

To my beautiful clients and friends who have trusted me as their coach and mentor on your hormone health and fertility journeys – your trust, vulnerability and transformation inspire me more than you know. You are the heartbeat behind this work.

To the mentors, teachers and practitioners who have shaped my understanding of the body, hormones and holistic health – thank you for sharing your wisdom and guidance. And to my coaches who guided me to move beyond fear, release old limitations and step fully into the role of creator in my own life – your support has given me the courage and clarity to share this work in my own unique way.

Thank you to the challenges and setbacks in life, especially the acne, which felt so painful and confidence-crushing at the time. Sometimes life's biggest challenges become our greatest blessings. For me, they led me to this book and the work I get to share with women.

To the wonderful team at Dean Publishing – thank you for helping make this book possible, for holding such a high vision for it, and for ensuring that my voice, story and message can reach the hands and hearts of as many women as possible.

And finally, to you – the reader. Thank you for choosing yourself. For choosing to learn about the incredible gift that is your menstrual cycle, to be empowered by it, and to live in alignment with it. I hope this book inspires you to nourish your body, honour your rhythms, and eat with the flow.

Thank you so much for supporting this book.

As a gift, I've created an exclusive bonus e-book with 24 additional recipes, just for you.

Scan the QR code to get instant access.

# REFERENCES

Baker JM, Al-Nakkashc L, Herbst-Kralovetza MM (2017) 'Estrogen–gut microbiome axis: Physiological and clinical implications', *Maturitas* 103: 45–53.

Battaglia S, Cozzi M, Ranieri FR, Gaio E, Benetti F and Curti V (2024) 'Effects of a Novel Combination of Magnesium, Tryptophan, Resveratrol, and Saffron on Oxidative Stress, Prostaglandin F2α, and Intracellular Ca2+ Levels in an In-vitro Model of Myometrium.' *Minerva Biotechnology and Biomolecular Research 35*(4). https://doi.org/10.23736/s2724-542x.23.02989-9.

Briden L (2018) *Period Repair Manual: Every woman's guide to better periods.* Macmillan Australia.

Brillhart MM, Gassen J, Lin L, Hugoboom G, Hugoboom B, and Hill S (2025) 'Does a menstrual cycle phase-based approach to fitness and nutrition improve outcomes for women? A study of 28 wellness users.' https://doi.org/10.31234/osf.io/39rwn_v1.

Brighton J (2020) *Beyond the Pill: A 30-Day Program to Balance Your Hormones, Reclaim Your Body, and Reverse the Dangerous Side Effects of the Birth Control Pill.* HarperCollins.

Chavarro JE, Willett WC, Skerrett PJ (2009) *The Fertility Diet: Groundbreaking research reveals natural ways to boost ovulation and improve your chances of getting pregnant.* McGraw-Hill.

Chocano-Bedoya PO, Manson JE, Hankinson SE, Johnson SR, Chasan-Taber L, Ronnenberg AG, Bigelow C and Bertone-Johnson ER (2013) 'Intake of Selected Minerals and Risk of Premenstrual Syndrome', *American Journal of Epidemiology 177*(10): 1118–27. https://doi.org/10.1093/aje/kws363.

Dullo P and Vedi N (2008) 'Changes in Serum Calcium, Magnesium and Inorganic Phosphorus Levels During Different Phases of the Menstrual Cycle', *Journal of Human Reproductive Sciences 1*(2): 77. https://doi.org/10.4103/0974-1208.44115.

Hay L (1984) *Heal Your Body: The mental causes for physical illness and the metaphysical way to overcome them.* Hay House.

Kapper C, Oppelt P, Ganhör C, Gyunesh AA, Arbeithuber B, Stelzl P and Rezk-Füreder M (2024) 'Minerals and the Menstrual Cycle: Impacts on Ovulation and Endometrial Health', *Nutrients 16*(7): 1008. https://doi.org/10.3390/nu16071008.

Kim K, Wactawski-Wende J, Michels KA, Schliep KC, Plowden TC, Chaljub EN and Mumford SL (2018) 'Dietary Minerals, Reproductive Hormone Levels and Sporadic Anovulation: Associations in Healthy Women With Regular Menstrual Cycles', *British Journal of Nutrition 120*(1): 81–89. https://doi.org/10.1017/s0007114518000818.

Kirkpatrick, B (2018) *Healthy Hormones: A practical guide to balancing your hormones.* Murdoch Books.

Raphael K (2021) *Microbiome Thyroid: Restore Your Gut and Heal Your Hidden Thyroid Disease.* Hachette.

Rubin LH and Marx BL (2012) 'Diminished Ovarian Reserve, Clomid, and Traditional Chinese Medicine: A Case Study', *Medical Acupunct 24*(4):273-280. https://doi.org/10.1089/acu.2012.0912.

Sharma N and Sharma A (2012) 'Thyroid profile in menstrual disorders', *JK Science 14*(1): 14-17.

Stevenson, S (2016) *Sleep Smarter: 21 essential strategies to sleep your way to a better body, better health and bigger success.* Hay House.

Thys-Jacobs S (2000) 'Micronutrients and the Premenstrual Syndrome: The Case for Calcium', *Journal of the American College of Nutrition 19*(2): 220–27. https://doi.org/10.1080/07315724.2000.10718920.

Todd A (2024) What's my body telling me: your body isn't the problem it's the solution. Dean Publishing

Vitti A (2020) *In the Flo: A 28 Day plan working with your monthly cycle to do more and stress less.* Harlequin.

Weschler T (2015) *Taking Charge of your fertility: The definitive guide to natural birth control, pregnancy achievement and reproductive health.* HarperCollins.

Yang T, Doherty J, Zhao B, Kinchla A, Clark JM and He L (2017) 'Effectiveness of Commercial and Homemade Washing Agents in Removing Pesticide Residues on and in Apples.' *Journal of Agricultural and Food Chemistry, 65*(44): 9744–9752. https://doi.org/10.1021/acs.jafc.7b03118.

www.ingramcontent.com/pod-product-compliance
Lightning Source LLC
Chambersburg PA
CBHW041602260326
41914CB00011B/1352